Humanitarian Solutions in the 21st Century

Series editor:
Larry Winter Roeder, Jr.

For further volumes:
http://www.springer.com/series/11580

Barbara Lucini

Disaster Resilience from a Sociological Perspective

Exploring Three Italian Earthquakes as Models for Disaster Resilience Planning

Springer

Barbara Lucini
Department of Sociology
Catholic University of Sacred Heart Milan
Milano, Italy

ISBN 978-3-319-04737-9 ISBN 978-3-319-04738-6 (eBook)
DOI 10.1007/978-3-319-04738-6
Springer Cham Heidelberg New York Dordrecht London

Library of Congress Control Number: 2014934299

Printed on acid-free paper

Springer is part of Springer Science+Business Media (www.springer.com)

Acknowledgements

I am grateful to all the people who made possible this research. Especially the people, of the National Civil Protection Service, for their availability; the personnel of the regions and municipalities; the experts interviewed; all the civil protection volunteers who participated in the survey; and all the ordinary people who told me of their dramatic experiences: I will never forget their eyes and what I saw in them.

I am grateful to my Tutors for the support, endurance, and patience they always has for me.

I am grateful to all the foreign professors, researchers, and students who were always available for suggestions and exchanges of ideas about my topic.

Finally, but just as important, I am grateful to all my Italian and foreign friends, who have always sustained me.

I am grateful to my beloved family, for my life, and for everything.

Contents

List of Figures

List of Tables

Chapter 1
Introduction

This work arises from sociological reflection about how people respond to and cope with a natural disaster. We live in a society where risks, disasters, and catastrophes are greatly increased because of a great number of new agents, in particular, the demographic explosion, better health conditions than in the past, the urbanization process, postindustrial dynamics at political as well as economic levels, new life styles, and, as a consequence, the difficulties of coordinating all these needs and social answers with the aim of improving living conditions for all the people in the world.

This new human situation can cause more risk and disasters than in past eras, before the industrialization process, for example, industrial risks and disasters such as those in Bhopal (1984) and Chernobyl (1989), to cite those that are more well-known; it is better not to forget the dramatic importance of natural disasters such as hurricanes, floods, earthquakes, such as those explored in this research in Italy: the Umbria–Marche earthquake in 1997; the Molise earthquake in 2002, and the Abruzzo earthquake in 2009.

For this reason, human and social discipline as sociology has many issues to point out in this discussion.

Comprehending which behaviors and responses are presented to face a disaster and, above all, understanding of the presence (or not) of sociological processes and actions of resilience is a topic for all those potentially at risk, such as ordinary people, volunteers, and public institutions and administrations, and it is the best way to try to improve shared knowledge about the disaster process, response, and possible prevention and planning activities.

The main questions used as background for this research are:

- What is disaster resilience from a sociological perspective and how can it be defined?
- How do people face a disaster and respond to it according to resilience dynamics from a sociological perspective?
- Can civil protection volunteers help the population affected by a disaster during this resilience process? If yes, during which specific disaster phases?

B. Lucini, *Disaster Resilience from a Sociological Perspective*, Humanitarian Solutions in the 21st Century, DOI 10.1007/978-3-319-04738-6_1,

– What kind of position do solidarity and conflict have within disaster resilience processes from a sociological point of view?

The aim of this research is to explore, through diverse theoretical and methodological instruments, the issues presented above and try to elaborate a definition of disaster resilience from a sociological perspective; to understand the social dynamics present within a disaster process; to comprehend the role (technical as well as supportive) of the Civil Protection Voluntary Service, considering that 2011 was the International Year of Voluntary Service; and to understand response to disaster and crisis situations by different agencies, both institutional and administrative, to underline the role of the civil society.

Specifically, this research starts with the theoretical background about the major theoretical proposals on these themes. In Chap. 2 an analysis of the literature about the sociological concepts of risk, vulnerability, emergency, disaster, and catastrophe is presented, with the aim of highlighting the social, symbolic, and anthropological implications in a disaster process; supposedly it is comprised of a number of interconnected phases—not by a linear logic but a circular one: mitigation, prevention, impact, response, reconstruction, and then back again to mitigation. Although this should be research from a sociological perspective and approach, it also is theoretically and methodologically useful to consider a historical approach to risk and disaster as well as an anthropological one.

After this necessary theoretical excursus, attention turns to the specific issue of resilience from a sociological perspective in the context of a natural disaster and the specific fieldwork for this research project: three Italian earthquakes.

Analyzing the use of the concept of resilience from other human and social sciences such as psychology and anthropology, I tried to understand the general theme, concepts, and implications necessary to articulate a sociological discourse on resilience within a natural disaster; in particular, in Chap. 3, a personal reflection on this issue is given, taking into consideration the main concepts of sociological origins, such as social capital, solidarity, altruism, and collective behavior, in the context of crises and disasters.

In Chap. 4 the civil protection system in Italy and its differences from the civil defense system are presented to understand the position of the civil protection volunteers within this organization and their potential for better disaster resilience.

The second and empirical part of this research focuses on the description of the three Italian earthquakes—Umbria–Marche (1997), Molise (2002), and Abruzzo (2009)—explored for this research. These three natural disasters were chosen because they represent three different "eras" of Italian civil protection organizations with cultural, political, economic, and social implications and because even if we refer to close geographical areas—Umbria in the central region and Abruzzo and Molise in the south of Italy—they have many differences regarding the responses by the population, public administrations, and civil protection volunteers.

The exploration of different social groups required the use of various methodological approaches and instruments typical of a mixed-methods approach. Chapter 4 presents information according to a second data analysis of such things as laws and other administrative documents applying to the Civil Protection Voluntary

Service and organizations in general, with the aim of showing the legislative and administrative context of the Italian Civil Protection Service and its evolution during the past 60 years.

Chapter 5 is focused on the description of the three earthquakes cosidered such as three fieldworks. It represents personal note by the researcher from the fieldworks, suggesting enlightenment ideas for the future analysis.

Chapter 6 analyzes the interviews collected from the civil protection experts on the issue of the Civil Protection Voluntary Service in an attempt to study and understand the role and implications of public administrations involved in natural disasters.

Chapter 7 represents the findings from the analysis of the national online questionnaire for civil protection volunteers, uploaded on the web site of the Itstime project by Catholic University of Sacred Heart—Milan and disseminated by mailing list at the local, provincial, regional, and national levels. This was necessary because of the impossibility of proceeding with a probabilistic sample due to the lack of any official list of civil protection voluntary organizations and groups.

Finally, Chap. 8 collects interviews with ordinary people through an ethnosociological approach to life stories and collecting the voices of those affected by earthquakes to comprehend the different and possible disaster resilience processes and their ties with the civil protection volunteers and civil society.

Listening to and understanding their voices had the advantage of comprehending the social and sociological resilience processes and dynamics and their presence or absence in a society and in a specific community beyond the importance of social relationships to cope with and face a disaster.

The three various methodological paths demonstrated were useful, considering that there are three main social actors involved in a natural disaster and the typical disaster response process.

I am referring to the three different methodological techniques and instruments related to the three social actors involved:

1. Interviews to the experts
2. online questionnaire for civil protection volunteers involved in the three earthquakes management
3. life story /recit de vie to ordinary peole

Some interesting findings are collected at the end of this book: a definition of disaster resilience from a sociological perspective, methodological reflections on the importance of an ethnographic approach to comprehend the experience lived by ordinary people, and the necessity of improving the social research instruments for civil protection volunteers.

In conclusion, this research demonstrates the importance of the civil society and the social relationships that take place during disasters or crises to enhance and make possible disaster resilience for the communities and societies stricken by them as well as the fundamental necessity of improving disaster resilience within the prevention actions, without forgetting that all the reflections and discussions on these issues are related to the more fundamental questions of democracy, security, safety, and human dignity.

Part I
Theoretical and Organizational Backgrounds

Chapter 2
Sociological Questions of Crises and Disasters in Our Contemporary Society

This chapter analyzes the evolution and theoretical changes of the fundamental sociological concepts of disaster, such as crisis, disaster, vulnerability, and risk. Crisis is considered within the social and cultural frameworks of our contemporary societies as are their characteristics of urgency, disruption, and complexity. Crisis shows the change of individual and social habits when people and communities are stricken by natural stress agents or those related to human activities.

Disaster is understood according to different traditional schools of thought and it is defined as the evidence of crisis and its consequences. The main theoretical background when considering the various definitions of disaster is represented by American, German, and Italian studies with their peculiarities in terms of disasters and their theoretical and methodological conceptualizations.

Another concept considered during the introduction of this research is vulnerability and its definition. In particular, the final aim of this research was to analyze and identify social vulnerability and its main features.

Related to the definition of vulnerability is the concept of risk and its evolution. A different definition of risk is presented, according to the necessity of the consideration of resilience as a basilar component of risk itself.

2.1 Which Crisis? Brief Overview of Definitions of *Crisis*

When we talk about crisis, the first thought on it is that it represents a moment of disruption, discontinuity, a specific time during which the previous competencies and knowledge are insignificant because of their meaningless congruence with an efficacious response that all systems in crisis require. According to Hermann (1972, quoted in Choi et al. 2010), *a crisis is a situation that incorporates the following three conditions: a surprise to decision makers, a threat to high-priority goals, and a restricted amount of time available for response.*

B. Lucini, *Disaster Resilience from a Sociological Perspective*, Humanitarian Solutions in the 21st Century, DOI 10.1007/978-3-319-04738-6_2,

In particular, crisis has been defined as a serious threat to the basic structures or the fundamental values and norms of a system, which under time pressure and highly uncertain circumstances necessitates making vital decisions (Rosenthal et al. 1989 quoted in Handbook of disaster Research 2006). A fundamental aspect of crisis is its disruption to organized time and its routine: *the crisis is logically constituted by routine, and its solution comes from external sources,*[1] *. . . and there is an asymmetry in the evaluation of crisis and routine* (Wagner 2004).

Specifically, crisis may be identified by three key components: threat, uncertainty, and urgency (Quarantelli et al. 2006). Recognizing the important role of each previous component in our societies and their implications within the crisis and disaster management process is the best way to learn, plan, and respond to a crisis situation. It is important to focus attention on the similarity of these three characteristics with the elements present in contemporary societies. In fact, actual societies, and in particular the urban social organization, can be comprehended through the same assumptions of crisis.

In current societies we find threats represented not only by natural agents (we intend natural agent to be understood as natural disasters such as earthquakes, hurricanes, tornados, floods, and so on) but also by a critical number of increasing technological and other threats caused by human actions or a system of concauses since the start of the industrial era.

Uncertainty is the other basilar characteristic of our societies and crisis itself. It is caused by great numbers of variables such as economic instability, political conflicts, environmental weaknesses, demographically unbalanced situations related to the macrovariables, wherever present, of globalization and immigration.

Urgency is another key word to define our present condition; we could refer to the nature of time *as a human condition characterized by time-binding and time-bound* (Bauman 1999). The sociologist Bauman also presents a specific definition of time in our era: *what is important is the speed not the duration* (Bauman 2006a, b).

So, time, in the form of urgency, is the last characteristic to introduce, in general terms, the question of crisis, but underneath this first concept we can also recognize that in a crisis and disaster process time, together with space, are the two systemic coordinates necessary to understand the process of a disaster and to plan prevention, response, and reconstruction activities. In particular, time compression is a specific element of a crisis.

The concept of time belongs to the anthropological and universal question of mankind in all eras and in all daily actions, but within a condition of crisis it assumes an important role (Clavandier 2004) because it represents a particular space, during which the actions of preventing, planning, and coping with a crisis take place. So, its functions are represented not only by a normative pattern (Pacelli and Marchetti 2007) but also other various types of time dimensions are considered (Elias 1986).

[1] Die Krise ist konstitutionlogisch betrachtet vor der Routine da; sie setzt eine Krisenloesung, die sich bewaehrt hat, immer schon voraus. (…) genau daraus leitet sich die Asymmetrie im Verhaeltnis von Krise und routine her.

Sociologically speaking, one of the first social considerations of crisis was the one proposed by Morin (1968, 1976), who explained a crisis as a concept at the macro level, where the complexity and uncertainty are the base and the approach is systemic, cybernetic, and neg-anthropic (Lombardi 2005).

The systemic level is represented by the presence of the aspects of diversity and similarity; within the cybernetics level the focus is on the dynamic equilibrium among different parts of the system, and the last level considers the inevitable process of disorganization in the system. In particular, the social disorder caused by a crisis could be seen as a phase during which established institutions lose their influence (Almond et al. 1973; Linz and Stepan; Zimmerman 1983).

Many sociological issues are part of this situation: the question of social order and disorder (Miller 2007), the functioning of public administrations, the competences of relief aid organizations, and the fundamental trust relationship between the population and the institutions. We can also speak about the power of legitimacy and democracy, which is hidden by these general issues.

This last concept refers to the final rights belonging to the population affected by a crisis to be an active part of the response, above all, but also before the event in the preventive phase, as well as playing a significant proactive role in the reconstruction period through a participative pattern. In this way, crisis determines a moment of social change within the organization of the community, city, or nation stricken by it: sometimes the impact of the crisis and the outcome of the disaster determine the complete change of social relationship and the previous social, economic, and political organization.

The possibility and the way to reconstruct after a crisis strictly depend on the model of crisis response and crisis management present in that specific country or community. The different kinds of activities and functions useful in responding to a crisis are determined by the specific model of organization and interpretation typical of each nation, country, city, or community stricken by a crisis. Considering this issue allows us to understand better the sociopsychological approach to a crisis, that is, comprehending individual and collective decision-making processes as a main aim of the discipline.

In particular, psychologists have done important research that helps us to understand the relation between human error, technology, organizational culture, and the development of a crisis. What is important to remember is the processes of amplification (Lombardi 1997a, b), sense making, and meaning making adopted and experienced by the population; according to Habermas (1975), *the crisis cannot be separated from the viewpoint of the one who is undergoing it*: crisis, like all the other concepts presented here, is a shared social construction and it needs adequate knowledge to detail this thinking and functionally respond to a crisis.

The amplification process is present in what has been called by Lombardi (2005) a crisis communication model or wave model that points out the following factors:

- Culture meaning
- Cognitive structure
- Institutional response

- Role of mass media communication
- Crisis perception and the possibility of preventing it
- Sense making by the population and all the different social groups affected by a crisis

So, if a crisis is considered a social and communication process, this model helps us to take into consideration the social perception and the role of crisis communication in the field of disaster management.

In the moment of crisis (Lagadec 1991, 1994), all we need is the possibility to return to normality or, better, to something we know and is familiar to us. This cognitive and social action requires a situation of trust in public institutions, cohesion, solidarity, altruism, and all other sorts of behaviors present during this situation; not only "positive" behaviors but also conflicts and discussions could take place and play a main role in these processes of trust negotiation and information sharing.

From a sociological point of view, the originality of the theory presented by Wagner (2004), based on an ideal type of crisis model related to structuralism and reflexivity principles, lies in the assumption of crisis as a socialization and dialectical process, where the popular and personal images of crisis have a crucial role in determining social behaviours, decision-making process, communication, and emergency planning.

When a crisis arises, according to the specific features of the systems, infrastructural organizations, and the population stricken by it, a disaster occurs. The following section is based on the different definitions of *disaster* and its sociological perspectives according to three orientations.

2.2 Disasters: Sociological Perspectives

What *disaster* and *catastrophe* mean from sociological and anthropological perspectives is not an innovative and postmodern question; instead their definitions have been a fundamental issue from the beginning of mankind. These matters are so basilar because they involve different and important aspects of human life (Gilbert 1995; Smith and Hoffman 1999, 2002), such as security and safety perceptions, familiar and emotional aspects, cognitive and cultural frameworks, organizational institutions, basic needs to survive, and anthropological wishes, for example, new experiences, identification, dominion, and security (Thomas and Znaniecki 1958 [1918/1920]).

In a situation of disaster, people could observe every kind of social implication and human relationship: the issue of control and disorder connected with legal and institutional aspects, solidarity, and altruism as sociopsychological implications during the initial impact and after the emergency; organizational factors related to the first responders; and crisis and disaster management strategies (Stallings and Quarantelli 1985). In general, disasters have been connected with the social change of the community stricken by these critical events.

According to sociological tradition, theories and reflections about what disaster is can be identified by referring to three different traditions and dimensions of disaster:

1. American studies
2. German studies
3. Italian studies

American studies based on the definition of disaster (Rodriguez, Quarantelli and Dynes 2006) are characterized by their attention on social disintegration, social change, and social disorders (Prince 1920). The first formal and social-scientific definition of disaster was elaborated by Fritz (1961 and then in 1968), who *saw disaster as an event impacting an entire society or some subdivision and including the notion of real impact with threat of impact but emphasized that essential functioning of the society is prevented* (1961, cited in Perry 2006). This is a "classical" period as defined by Perry (2006), and it represents the time from after the Second World War until 1961, with the definition by Fritz.

In this framework, the primary group of sociological thoughts about disasters (Quarantelli 1978, 1982, 1990, 1993, 1995) take into consideration the role of the social norm paradigm, the system of social norms in which all people live and the question of social change at a macro level (Quarantelli and Davis 2011). The attention in this period was focused on the social order, and from a systemic view, a disaster was seen as an element of disruption and destruction of the previous order and all its established components, which constituted a society.

According to this approach, a disaster represents a sociological thinking through of different levels of a society:

- At a microsociological level, we can conceptualize this issue as connected with cultural skills, personal behaviors, preventive and response activities, individual vulnerability, training activities, and pattern of general resources (economic, cultural, social, organizational).
- At a mesosociological level, as considered by Merton (1949) and his theoretical proposal.
- We can consider the family behavior adopted before and during a disaster situation as well as the actions at the community and societal levels, which are characterized by different and peculiar features.
- At a macrosociological level we consider, as mentioned earlier, the general assessment of a society and, in our contemporary societies, globalization activities in terms of preventing, coping with, and response to a disaster, with reference to the "global community" by Bauman (2001).

Coming back to the social definition of a disaster, citing Perry and his analysis (2006), we need to show the definition by Barton (1963), who *saw disaster as one collective stress situation arising when members of a social system fail to receive expected conditions of life from the system.*

Finally, it is fundamental to consider the crucial definition of disaster from a sociological perspective as elaborated by Quarantelli (2000), as cited in Perry (2006):

He (Quarantelli 2000, p. 682) identifies disasters in terms of a variety of defining features. They: (1) are sudden-onset occasions, (2) seriously disrupt the routines of collective units, (3) cause the adoption of unplanned courses of action to adjust to the disruption, (4) have unexpected life histories designated in social space and time and (5) pose danger to valued social objects.

He subsequently emphasized that a disaster represents vulnerability, reflecting weakness in social structure or social system (Quarantelli 2005, p. 345)

This definition considers various aspects of disasters and highlights the importance of unplanned actions that cause social disorder and stop the communication and relational systems of a society stricken by it.

American studies, in the framework of the sociology of disaster, are basilar elements to comprehend better the tie between sociological tradition and its themes as well as practical and operative tools in risk communication, crisis and disaster management, and organized emergency response.

According to this perspective and the aim of this general overview, another consideration should be made for the German tradition of disaster studies (Dombrowsky 1981, 1989; Jaeger 1977; Japp 1996, 2000, 2003; Plate and Merz 2001; Clausen et al. 2003; Pfister and Summematter 2004; Felgentreff and Glade 2008; Hammerl et al. 2009; Voss and Wagner 2010), which is historically related to the lack of language distinction between a disaster and a catastrophe: referring to cultural and social levels, it is quite interestingly observed that, in German, there is only the term *catastrophe* to refer at the same time to either a disaster or a catastrophe. This means that not only is attention paid to the level of damage as a consequence of disaster itself but also the focus is on the social aspects that a disaster manifests.

Clausen and Jaeger (1975) defined disasters as *the results of the fact that social secrets were continually produced. If dangers did not have secret causes, then the lightning could have struck out of the blue*; Clausen et al. (1978) state that *disasters are thus a normal (and often highly revealing) component of the social systems themselves, this depends on the regularity with which antagonisms in a particular society allow knowledge to different classes or groups*.

In the 1994, Clausen elaborated another definition of disaster, as follows: "it is as an extra accident that it is analysed at social level, as an alternative to something considered normal."[2] Disaster, through German tradition, is also understood as a socially constructed process[3] characterized, not always but often, by conflicting actions and their ritual circles, which oriented the social construction itself (Clausen 1994). Clausen elaborated his macrosociological model of the disaster process (1992): in the German language, it is called the FAKKEL model, whereas the English translation is the PERDUE Model, which is an acronym for:

- P: peace
- E: everyday routine
- R: a hidden, radical element enters

[2] Translation from the original German language by the author: "Die Katastrophe ist als ein Extremfall der moeglichen Veflechtungen anlysierbar, insoweit: immer etwas Normales."

[3] This vision is influenced by the times in which it was first thought and by the theoretical identification of social problems as a product of a process of collective definitions (Blumer 1970).

- D: disaster strikes—social
- U: unconditional surrender of collective defence—neither professional elites nor power elites nor other ruling classes
- E: evaporation of all value systems destroys institutional beliefs, ideologies, and religions, and the secular rationality of imminent danger prevails.

Dombrowsky (1981, 1989), in his general elaboration of the theoretical definition of disaster as a social construction, identifies three characteristics of disaster[4]: (1) disaster as metaphor; (2) disaster as imagination; and (3) disaster as causality. The presence of metaphor and imagination are typical features of German philosophy and social theorization. Furthermore, this aspect underlines the possibility of including sociological and anthropological elements in the discussion of disaster and its definition, elements useful for focusing attention on the social process of the disaster itself.

Another model for the explanation of the disaster process, called LIPDAR, was elaborated by Dombrowsky and Clausen (1983). Per the Economy-point.org website[5]: it is an acronym for five distinctive and discreet phases and from the operational sequence of disaster process development. *The phases are:*

1. *the latency phase: a threatening damage event is possible*
2. *the identification phase: the warnings identify the type of disaster*
3. *the definition phase: when the occurring danger is categorized, the social positions (competencies), which can be ready, are concomitantly defined and assigned responsibilities*
4. *the personalization phase: sociologically this is the most important phase; "rescuers" and "victims" (ev. already "authors") are identified for action and assigned them; also, rule-relevant social roles in addition their expected roles (e.g., determination, courage, authority and/or self-protection, following SAMness) are activated; "outstanding ones" are categorized (e.g., "gaffer")*
5. *the action phase: when a disaster is fought, prevented, and/or gelindert ("employment"); fall of the victims and rescuers is not impossible*
6. *the feedback phase: criticism, things learned, and prophylaxis for the survivors of participants or others are formulated and organized if necessary*

> LIPDAR is to be differentiated from FAKKEL, a more long-term expiration operational sequence that starts from the earliest stages of a disaster's genesis through to its late phases. (Clausen and Dombrowsky 1983).

Although it is quite difficult to use these two models, or even one of them, for methodological and operative proposals, they assume real importance in the definition of a disaster from a sociological approach. Instead, a useful distinctive classification of disaster's definition according to German authors, and the context within which the disaster should be studied (even if the destructive elements of disruption, damage, and loss are always present), can be the following (Geenen 2008):

- Disaster definition in analytical convergence with social disaster (Katastrophendefinition in analytischer Annaeherung—Sozialkatastrophe)

---

[4] Katastrophen als Metaphor; Katastrophen als Imagination; Katastrophen als Kausalitaet.

[5] http://www.economypoint.org/l/lidpar.html.

- Disaster definition on the basis of grades of sadness and coping with the difficulties (Katastrophendefintion auf der Grundlage des Grades der Betroffenheit und Bewaeltigungfaehigkeit)
- Disaster definition based on damage (Katastrophendefintion basierend auf der Schadenshoehe)
- Disaster definition based on operational aspects (Katastrophendefintion basierend auf Operationalisierungsaspekten)

An interesting actual approach is presented by Voss (2010), considering the work done by Fischer (2003).

As cited by Voss (2010), Fisher *proposed the establishment of a classification system for catastrophes similar to the Richter scale for earthquakes. Fischer advocates a distinction between the Disaster as a precipitating event resulting in widespread destruction and distress and the Sociology of Disasters which addresses the process of change from daily routine to the emergence of a (usually) temporary alternative and again all attained information is distributed on a scale involving ten categories: (1) everyday emergencies, (2) severe emergencies, (3) partial disruption and adjustment in a town, township or rural area, (4) massive disruption and adjustment in a town, township or rural area, (5) partial disruption and adjustment in a small or medium city, (6) massive disruption and adjustment in a small or medium city, (7) partial disruption and adjustment in a large city, (8) massive disruption and adjustment in a large city, (9) catastrophic and/or simultaneous massive disruption and adjustment in several communities, (10) the complete annihilation of a society.*

This represents one of the most complete definitions of disaster because of its consideration of the various aspects included in a disaster concept.

Furthermore, focusing attention on Italian studies and their definition of disaster, I present a brief overview of Italian disaster and crisis studies because of their discontinuity and their lack of strong theoretical and methodological corpus after the 1990s. Specifically, Italian studies focused on the crisis and emergency process as well as risk communication and perception.

However, historically speaking, Italian studies should refer to the ISIG Centre, Institute of International Sociology Gorizia, held in Gorizia during the 1980s, and their vision of disaster is based on sociotechnical and sociosystemic perspectives connected with a sociological vision but also is related to a multidisciplinary approach, taking into account, for example, the psychological and technical features of crises and disasters.

Nowadays, this research center is interested in the social dynamics that are part of the disaster process. It focuses attention on environmental planning, environmental risk and its governance, sustainability, risk communication, vulnerability, and resilience from a cognitive and structural viewpoint.

As always, in Italy, the first structural studies took place after the big disasters in the 1980s (floods and earthquakes) and were authored by Pelanda, Strassoldo, Cattarinussi, and De Marchi. During the 1980s and 1990s (Cattarinussi and Pelanda 1981; De Marchi et al. 2001), there was a collaboration between the Italian authors and E.L. Quarantelli

(Quarantelli et al. 1981), but then their research paths were different and the Italian authors chose a different approach in the study of disasters and calamities.

Another Italian research center on crises, disasters, and emergencies is ITSTIME, Italian Team for Security, Terrorist Issues and Managing Emergencies based at the Department of Sociology, Catholic University, Milan. A specific research project is IDRA, Itstime Disaster Resilience Agency, aimed at being a point of reference for future reflections and research projects on the issues of disaster resilience and its correlated themes, risk and disaster management and crisis response.

2.3 Addressing Risks from a Sociological Perspective

Risks of various types (Adam et al. 2000; Beck 1992, 2001, 2003) have always been presented throughout the history of mankind. Before industrialization the typical risks were natural ones (Beato 1998), but after this period, and in the new era, types of risk have been implemented with technological risk and terrorist attack according to sociopolitical perspectives (Beck 1986).

As Bauman (2000) said, *risk is a constant of human life*[6]; further, as Lombardi (2005) pointed out: *in this process risk seems not determinate from external conditions* (external risk), but risk is determined by the decision making process.[7] For a period of time we have believed that technological inventions (Alexander 2000) and their new implications can be useful to protect our lives from hazard and risk; instead, it has never been so.

At an institutional level, as represented by International Strategy for Disaster Reduction of the United Nations (UNISDR), risk is defined as *the probability of harmful consequences, or expected losses (deaths, injuries, property, livelihoods, economic activity, disruption or environment damage) resulting from the interaction between natural or human-induced hazards and vulnerable conditions.*

Starting with the historical introduction of the term *risk*, we note that its use is quite recent in terms of eras. In fact, its first use can be recalled within the context of gambling and correlated with sea voyages during the 12th and 13th centuries and its social and symbolic representation. As terminology, the word *risk* is difficult to present because of its different possible origins, such as Arabian, Latin, or Greek.

Luhmann (1991, 1993) places the use of this word in the phase between the last Middle Age and the first Modern Age; in this period the word is used to indicate a possibility of choice and, eventually, its worst effects.

The evolution of this concept is based on the new reflection about the role of nature, God, and destiny, which can be the cause of something dangerous (Luhmann 1991). Thus it seems a "naturalist" conception of risk correlated with the assumption of nature as both a good and bad element at the same time (Walter 2009).

---

[6] Bauman (2000): "il rischio è una costante delle vita umana".

[7] Lombardi (2005): "in questo processo il rischio non appare più determinato da condizioni esterne all'individuo (rischio esterno), ma determinato al rischio inerente ai meccanismi di presa di decisione (rischio interno)".

A change in this conceptualization was made possible with the coming of probabilistic calculation and the introduction of a deterministic approach to social and human life (Kaplan and Garrick 1981; Lash 2000). With this definition, in fact, it is possible to know, anticipate, and foresee many elements present in human daily life and, in this way, improve the quality of life. This perspective has been present during Enlightenment, along with the characteristics of rationality and power referring to cultural, political, and economic beliefs.

In particular, attention was focused on the difference attitudes confronting the position of homo faber and self-made man: two typical concepts of English and American cultures. The basilar assumption here is the possibility of every single man to be a protagonist and participating actor in his own destiny and fortune. In this context the deterministic and positivistic approach arose, which was pervasive for a long period of time. In 1921, Knight introduced, for the first time, made a distinction between risk and uncertainty, referring to the probabilistic quantification that is possible for the first concept but not for the second.

In general, historically speaking, the term *risk* had its origin in the economic context, where the fundamental question was about the calculation of the advantages or disadvantages typical of a social scenario. The history of the studies about the concept of risk correlated to a rational logic started in the years between 1948 and 1953. Specifically, the book *The Theory of Games* by von Neumann and Morgenstern permitted the start of elaborate scientific and empirical studies of risk. The term *risk* also introduces a distinction from the term *hazard*: the latter is considered as a potential threat, whereas *risk* is the probability of the presence of an hazard (Walter 2008). In this period, risk was defined as the product of damage associated with a critical event and the probability that this event has to occur.

The calculation of risk can be presented as $D \times P/T$, where D is damage, P is probability, and T represents time. What has been noted with this definition (Lombardi 2005) is the linear relation between damage and intensity; however; it is not possible for it to be a linear relation because of the introduction of the element of vulnerability.

So, the redefinition of risk (Lombardi 2005) is the product of a probabilistic value and intensity value, the probability that the event occurs to which is added the vulnerability[8]:

$$\text{Risk} = P \times I \times V,$$

Where P is probability, I is intensity, and V is vulnerability. The assumption is that probability and intensity are characteristics of the stressor, whereas vulnerability belongs to the victim and to the system potentially at risk. This consideration is important in terms of prevention and planning activities, as shown by Phillips et al. (2010) and Enarson (2007).

Vulnerability also appears in the definition of risk elaborated by Schneiderbauer and Ehrlich (cited in Birkmann 2006): *$Rah = Hah \times Ea \times Vah$, where h relates to the type of hazard (determined in its severity and its temporal extent); a is the*

[8]A specific paragraph about the concept of vulnerability and, in particular for my aims, social vulnerability follows.

geographical region affected by hazard h, E is the exposure, and V is vulnerability, such as people's ability to cope with hazard h in area a.

Other aspects to be considered in the development of this research is the geographical and social context in which a risk or critical event could be present. It is important to consider the different needs and their implications according to the spatial definition, with the aim of orienting possible responses to the risk in terms of prevention and preparedness (Denney 2005).

To understand better the social theories elaborated during the past 30 years, it seems to be a useful decision to propose the classification elaborated by Renn (1992), where the study of risk has been correlated with the following main arguments:

- Study that is oriented on the organizational aspects of risk (Perrow 1984; Clarke 1989)
- Study of the context of the sociology of disaster (Dynes et al. 1987)
- Analysis of mass media and risk communication (Mazur 1981; Lichtenberg and MacLean 1991; Peltu 1988; Stallings 1990; Peters et al. 1997; Lombardi 2005)
- Risk conflicts and their causes (O'Riodan et al. 1997; von Winterfeldt and Edwards 1984; Edwars and von Winterfeldt 1986; Dietz et al. 1989)
- Analysis of equity and lack of correctness (Kasperson and Kasperson 1983; MacLean 1986; Rosa 1998)
- Analysis of risk distribution among classes and populations (Schnaiberg 1980; Beck 1986)
- Study regarding epistemology and legitimization of knowledge of risk (Rip 1985; Jasanoff 1986; Dietz and Rycroft 1987; Evers and Nowotny 1987)

In this specific work, the concept of risk is considered in the field of the sociology of disaster according to different traditions of thinking and, considering the importance of such studies for the risk perception and the social dynamics, which are the basis for adequate and effective prevention and planning activities, to potential risk for the population living in a specific social space (Krimsky and Golding 1992).

What has been said before can be reconsidered in the field of risk analysis and the many perspectives within it (as shown by Marinelli [1993]). These included the following items.

- The origin of risk analysis can be found in engineering perspectives; the first method used was elaborated by Starr (1969) and called "revealed preferences." It was based on the calculation of advantage and disadvantage and focused on econometric studies. The point was on the possibility of finding a compromise between the needs of the population and the economic and political context.
- Another perspective was presented by Formal Analysis and underlines the fact that each process of risk construction is a decisional process. In this context what is more important is the decisions made by the populations and institutions in a potential risk area.

- Psychological and psychometric perspectives (Tversky and Kahneman 1974; Lichtenstein 1978; Kasperson 1988; Slovic 1985) were based on the key concept of risk perception and its influence in the decisional process and within all phases constituting the management of risk, crisis, and disaster.
- The key argument of the decisional analysis perspective was the effort to change uncertainty into probability to allow a possible social and technological control of risk in a society.
- Cost-benefit analysis, or risk benefit analysis, and its assumption is the calculation of advantages and disadvantages for all people involved in a possible risk process.
- Decision analysis is useful, methodological speaking, for the decisional process and its related actions in conditions of uncertainty.
- The last one is represented by what is called cultural theory, and Douglas and Wildavsky (1982) are the major authors of it (Douglas 1991, 1996). Their proposal also is known as social construction of risk and the scheme of grid and group. The first represents the dimension of social differentiation and the intensity of institutional interaction, whereas the second refers to the level of boundaries between different social groups.

Crossing these two dimensions, Douglas and Wildavsky (1982) identified four positions:

- Individualist: weak grid, weak group
- Atomize subordination: strong grid, weak group
- Hierarchic: strong grid, strong group
- Sectarian: weak grid, strong group

This represented a new proposal to study and understand the concept of risk and its presence in our societies. Even if their efforts to structure another theory on the concept of risk and the attention paid to the social group present in a society potentially at risk, they received some critiques about the theoretical formulation and its schematic and, for some aspects, the almost "deterministic" approach if applied to our complex societies and all their shades (Marinelli 1993). What could be important in this theory is the focus on social aspects and social interactions, which are part of the general social construction of risk. In fact, when referring to the concept of risk we may consider two positions that are not opposite but interconnected: One refers to risk as a product of natural hazards or technological hazards caused by human actions, as shown earlier. The other refers to the concept of risk considering attention on social construction and the social perception of risk. With this background, risk is a shared and building concept made up by all the social groups present in a society or community.

An interesting classification of risk is presented by Lombardi (2005), who identifies natural risk and social risk. The first concept may be passive or active. Passive risks do not have a specific objective, for example, earthquakes and floods. Active risks present a basilar norm of occurrence, for example, an epidemic.

The second concept may be intended or unintended; this classification is made possible according to personal analysis in term of costs and benefits.

This general classification is followed by the identification of main variables (personally translated by the author) for the perception of risk collocated on a continuum (Lombardi 2005):

- Controlled–uncontrolled
- Known–unknown
- Frightful–not frightful
- Immediate–postponed
- Latent–present
- Specific–nonspecific
- Retrievable–irreversible

These factors seem to be the most important elements to orient and direct the perception of risk by a population potentially or not at risk, and they appear in different ways for mass media, the population, and institutions or public administrations. In fact, *the framework seeks to explain the apparent paradox that minor risks are often treated with great concern by the public, while other seemingly greater risks are ignored* (Krimsky and Golding 1992).

Another risk classification has been presented by Lupton (2002) and considers the specific contexts in which the risk could be manifest, such as:

- Risk of style of life
- Economic risk
- Criminal risk
- Health risk
- Social relations risk
- Environmental risk

This typology is useful to understand the role of context as a social space within which a risk could occur, and this theoretical framework underlines that *nothing is a risk in itself but it is a contingent product of historically, socially and politically created ways of seeing* (Lupton 1999).

The research done in Italy by Savadori et al. (1998) has taken into consideration two fundamental factors of risk: terrified risk and unknown risk. This theorization reflects two aspects elaborated by Yates and Stone (1992), which are the base for a "new" definition of risk including subjective parameters such as the meaning and the uncertainty of loss. What is important to underline with these theories is the different approaches of and comprehension of the phenomenon of risk.

The risk perception approach focuses attention on the personal, cultural, and social attitudes in understanding risk situations and conditions. This perspective is useful not only for psychologists but also to sociologists because of the focus on beliefs and attitudes belonging to people—and not only the rational side of a population (Weber 1981; Coleman 1990).

The main sociological aspect is the possible social control of risk and risk situations and the rationality attributed to disaster managers, volunteers, and public institutions who are responsible for crisis and disaster management. It could be argued that the consideration of a new paradigm, meaning risk as a social science question, has caused other social implications for all people involved in crisis and disaster process to arise.

Perception of risk has become a social component to take into account because of its importance in determining the psychological and mental imagination of risk and its practical implications for preventive and planning activities (Savadori et al. 1998). Therefore, risk is not only a social process but also a communication process (Scanlon 1982; Lombardi 2005).

This approach recognizes that risk is not only perceived and experienced by the population and public officers or risk managers. Instead it involves a great number of other people in what has been called mass media. The role of mass media (Scanlon 1982; Lombardi 2005) in a risk context considers all phases of the risk process:

- Prevention phase in the form of information for potential people at risk or vulnerable groups
- During the impact of risk to alert and help in crisis management
- After impact to communicate about and reflect on the crisis

The communication process is the basis for all other kinds of relationships and social changes (Mead 1966). Its characteristics allow us to share arguments, opinions, and ideas that are important to model our own response in the face of a risk, crisis, or disaster. In this process all elements of socialization are present:

- The sense of belonging (Falck 1994) to a community or a shared social space
- The sense of social and personal identity related to a community or social space
- Sharing social relationships, common values, beliefs and attitudes, and trust, which are fundamental in the perception of risk and the process of its acceptance

As we have seen previously, risk can be considered and represented as a social construction as well as a disaster (Clausen 1992). Another key element present in the definition of *disaster* (Lombardi 2005) is vulnerability: to understand what we call "vulnerability" and its components, especially social components, is the next aim.

2.4 Vulnerability

In line with the previous introduction and the ideas expressed about the change of society, our lifestyles, and the phenomena of globalization and urbanization, we indeed seem to have entered a "risk society" (Beck 1986). The awareness of being vulnerable and living in a vulnerable context is one of the first principles used to highlight the perception of risk and disaster as experienced by the population that was affected by three earthquakes in Italy. The perception of risk has the function of increasing or decreasing vulnerability, which becomes a strong element for the possibility of people to cope with and face up to a potential disaster (Alexander 1993). Risk perception also is based on many variables and indicators that are typical of individuals, organizations, populations, social groups, and institutional administrations. For this reason, vulnerability is a core component of the concept of risk. In some aspects, prior knowledge of the potential risk and exposure to that risk by the population have provided an opportunity to understand better the components of vulnerability (Heijmans 2001; Levine 2004) within a social context.

According to Boin and 't Hart (2006), *the causes of vulnerability often reside deep within the system.* For this reason, the first task within this theoretical reflection is to highlight the specific sociological context to which it refers. In fact, as Pelanda wrote (1981), *even though many of these definitions stress the socio-ecological quality of the term vulnerability, they assume a relative independence between the probability of occurrence of a destructive event and the sociological context.* This is typical of the history of studies about vulnerability and is connected with the historical period during which they have taken place.

The sociosystemic view underlines the lack of technical preparedness and focuses attention on the technologies in the field of preventive training and improvement of technical progress. This was expressed well by Quarantelli and Tierney (1979): *the community preparedness necessitates social change, not mere technological upgrading.*

In general terms, the literature about vulnerability presents *25 different definitions, concepts, and methods to systematise vulnerability* (Birkmann 2006). As cited by Birkmann and Bogardi (2004), there is a sort of "confusion" about the definitions of vulnerability and the methodological implications of evaluating it and planning serviceable prevention activities. I give some definitions of vulnerability that outline some important aspects of this research.

Birkmann (2006), as cited by Schneiderbauer and Ehrilich (2004), pointed out that "vulnerability is a concept that evolved out of the social sciences and was introduced as a response to the purely hazard-oriented perception of disaster risk in the 1970s. Since the 1980s, the dominance of hazard-oriented prediction strategies based on technical interventions has been increasingly challenged by the alternative paradigm of using vulnerability as the starting point for risk reduction."

Vulnerability, according to Wisner et al. (2004), is *the characteristics of a person or group and their situation that influence their capacity to anticipate, cope with, resist and recover from the impact of a natural hazard (an extreme natural event or process).* Vulnerability is defined by Pelling (2003) as something that *denotes exposure to risk and the inability to avoid or absorb potential harm and vulnerability is broken down into three components: exposure, resistance and resilience.*

It is important to consider the context within which vulnerability is its own component. In particular, in the past 15–20 years, changes due to new ways of urbanization and the development of megacities (Koetter 2004) have radically changed the perception of risk and the awareness of vulnerability by populations. This kind of vulnerability seems to be more connected to political ecology than a systemic approach (Phillips et al. 2010).

Considering vulnerability from a systemic point of view allows us to take into consideration different components of systems and societies, their characteristics, their influences, and their implications within vulnerable contexts and different types of places. Space and place have a central role in this discussion to understand vulnerability from an ecological and spatial perspective as related to the anthropological sense and culture making, in particular, spatial vulnerability, which is *derived from physical space (location and the built environment)* (Waugh and Tierney 2007).

Vulnerability was defined by Wisner et al. (2004) as *the characteristics of a person or a group and their situation that influence their capacity to anticipate, cope with, resist and recover from the impact of a natural hazard (an extreme natural event or process)*. Vulnerability is a multidimensional concept and is characterized by different dimensions (Wilches and Chaux 1993): physical, economic, social, educational, political, institutional, cultural, environmental, and ideological. Furthermore, Villagràn de Leon (2001) identified components related to vulnerability: structural, functional, economic, human condition/gender, administrative, and environmental.

Villagràn de Leon (2004) also connects vulnerability within a risk and hazard context and uses this to define the triangle of risk and its three components: vulnerability, hazard, and deficiencies in preparedness. For him, vulnerabilities are (as cited in Birkmann 2006): *the pre-existing conditions that make infrastructures, processes, services and productivity more prone to be affected by an external hazard.*

As previously noted, vulnerability presents many dimensions considering its components and its conditions of origin. The categorization related to this issue has been elaborated by McEntire (2001), as cited in Ginige et al. (2009): "McEntire (2001) categorizes the variables, which interact to produce a future of increased vulnerabilities under physical, social, cultural, political, economic, and technological headings as given in the following list. This classification splits the social vulnerability in the earlier categorization into three separate groups as social, cultural and political dimensions of vulnerabilities. In addition, the environmental dimensions are brought under the physical variables here in contrast to the earlier division: physical, social, cultural, political, economic and technological."

Taking into account all the dimensions of vulnerability (Di Sopra and Pelanda 1984) is the first aim in the field of risk reduction and crisis and disaster management. Vulnerability appears as a basilar concept that allows us to understand the possibility of coping with risks and disasters, even if there is a need to clarify the position of vulnerability connected with resilience. In this practical field we focused on the opportunity to enhance the model of response by public institutions and volunteers, in particular with regard to prevention activities.

Before knowing the vulnerability of a system, a society, or a community, it is important to point out that what would be interesting is comprehending the level of awareness about its own vulnerability. In this specific context, the level of awareness refers to the difference between being vulnerable and being conscious of the vulnerability. As previously shown with the concept of risk, vulnerability also seems, as a whole, to be divided into two categories: concrete and practical vulnerability and the perception of vulnerability.

In many cases, for example, people exposed to hurricanes, earthquakes, and general natural disasters seem to be more aware of their vulnerable condition than those who are exposed to industrial, technical, or terrorist attacks. In this analysis it could be useful to take into consideration the role of tradition, the exchange of information, and basilar communication about the situation, the system, and environmental conditions. Interesting studies in this field could analyzing the role of the inter- and intragenerational passing on of rules and stories about vulnerable lifestyles.

Here, and for all other key concepts present in this work, the importance of social and communication processes appear clearly, and those things enhance the response to a crisis, prevention activities, and the social resilience process during and after a disaster.

Another question that is valid for all the theoretical concepts of risk, crisis, and disaster is their "double face" in terms of their understanding by and implications to public administrators, disaster managers, and mass media on the one hand, and the perception of the population and their behavior according to what they consider risky or vulnerable conditions and disaster on the other.

Moving along this continuum, the real challenge is represented by the improvement of emergency plans and the communication of prevention activities in the field of crisis and disaster management. In fact, in the middle of this continuum lies the possibility to understand and cope with risk, crisis, and disaster in the best way possible. In these actions the role of sociology is basilar to knowing and communicating the feelings of the population, which are fundamental in planning actions.

This double face is also a characteristic of vulnerability from a theoretical point of view and is expressed by Bohle (2001, cited in Birkmann 2006) as an external and internal side of vulnerability: *The internal side, coping, relates to the capacity to anticipate, cope with, resist, recover from the impact of a hazard; in contrast, the external side involves exposure to risks and shocks.* Again, *in social science the distinction between the exposure to external threats and the ability to cope with them is often used to underline the double structure of vulnerability* (van Dillen 2004). Because of the importance of time in risk and crisis situations, it is better to clarify the role of simultaneity when referring to these two sides of vulnerability and their mutual influence (Birkmann 2006).

2.4.1 Social Vulnerability

As we have previously shown, vulnerability is a multidimensional concept because of its qualitative characteristics. It is important to clarify vulnerability as related to this research and the choice to focus on a specific vulnerability: social vulnerability. The sociological approach to vulnerability should refer to social vulnerability because of its nature. The components of social vulnerability belong, in a strong way, to social process and sociological analysis.

Social vulnerability, as a general concept of vulnerability, has had many definitions during decades of study and research. Cannon et al. (2003), as cited in Birkmann (2006), *argue that social vulnerability is much more than the likelihood of buildings collapsing and infrastructure being damaged. Social vulnerability is a set of characteristics that include a person's:*

- *Initial well being*
- *Livelihood and resilience*
- *Self-protection*
- *Social protection*
- *Social and political networks and institutions*

This definition is very important in this context because it underlines aspects of vulnerability that are not directly related to technical and instrumental components. Instead it bases the assumption on the fact that *vulnerability is only partially determined by the type of hazard* (Cannon et al. 2003).

As cited in Birkmann (2006), Downing et al. (2006) *define six attributes to characterise social vulnerability based on the experiences of over two decades of research on this topic. They emphasise that social vulnerability is:*

- *The differential exposure to stress experienced or anticipated by the different units exposed*
- *A dynamic process*
- *Rooted in the actions and multiple attributes of human actors*
- *Often determined by social networks, economic, political and environmental interactions*
- *Manifested simultaneously on more than one scale*
- *Influenced and driven by multiple stresses*

The originality of sociological contributions is constituted by the importance of social networks and the possibility of analyzing and improving the resilient process that lies within them. The social levels of vulnerability could be identified as (Schneiderbauer and Ehrlich 2006):

- Individual
- Household
- Administrative community
- Cultural community
- National
- Regional

The focus here is on the contexts within which vulnerability can be present. As Villagràn De Leon said (cited in Birkmann 2006), "in the context of natural disasters, vulnerability can be associated with the predisposition of a system, a process, an institution, a community or a country to be affected when a natural event manifests itself."

A systematic analysis of the literature allow us to classify contexts used by various authors when defining the nature of vulnerability. These include:

- *the particular state of a system before an event triggers a disaster, described in terms of particular indicators or parameters of such a system;*
- *the probability of the outcome of the system, expressed in terms of losses, measured in terms of either fatalities or economic impact; and*
- *a combination of a particular state of the system with other factors such as the inherent capacity to resist the impact of the event (resilience) and the capacity to cope with it (coping capacities).*

From a sociological point of view, this means that it is necessary to rethink the social aspects involved in the vulnerability process and risks. Attention should be paid to the empowerment of social networks and their efficacy in the flow of, for example, communication and prevention information, or, more could be done to encourage people and groups to take an active role in a crisis.

Attention on the alternative perspectives of social vulnerability focuses on the dominant view of hazard and vulnerability and the vulnerability view (Enarson 2006, 2007). Specifically, Enarson proposed that the dominant view is characterized by:

- The physical processes of a hazard
- Management style emphasizes problem solving through hierarchies and authorities
- A top-down approach
- The use of technology, engineering, and science to address the hazard
- The goal of reducing physical damage
- The general philosophical approach being utilitarian and the conquest of nature
- The emphasis of bounded systems

Instead, the vulnerability view is characterized by:

- Addressing socioeconomic and political influences
- A management style emphasizing a decentralized approach that involves community-based problem solving
- A grassroots or bottom-up approach
- Using local knowledge, networks, imagination, and creativity to address the hazard
- The goal of reducing the social vulnerability of people
- The general philosophical approach being an equitable approach to reduce vulnerability and to work in concert with nature
- Emphasizing an open system and complexity

In this context I am trying to overcome the opposite and dialectical positions between the concept of vulnerability presented as a "dominant view" (Phillips et al. 2010) and the new one in which vulnerability is assumed to be a core element in disaster risk reduction studies. From a sociological position, it is more important to elaborate useful concepts and indicators taken from all the existing theories, including historical, social, geographical, political, and economic conditions, with the aim of presenting a new "dialectical proposal."

The present intent, given the main topics of resilience and disaster, is to put forward an approach that vulnerability is another side – although not the opposite – of resilience: *social vulnerability is not inevitably synonymous with lack of resilience* (Waugh and Tierney 2007). In fact, hazard and vulnerability, even if they belong to different perspectives, are crucial aspects of a disaster risk reduction discussion. They are two elements that cannot be separated or comprehended as only one thing without the other. This theoretical position is well expressed by Phillips et al. (2010): *from the vulnerability perspectives, it is necessary to understand both the physical impact of disasters and the social conditions that underline different outcomes.*

In planning activities and during the prevention and mitigation phases we need both of these approaches: the dominant view to understand better the types of hazard and technologies we can use in case of risk, crisis, or disaster and the vulnerability view to gain more knowledge about the characteristics of the population potentially at risk of or affected by disaster.

Developing the analysis and exploration of the coping mechanism model (Blaikie et al. 1994) allows us to understand the possibility of enhancing our safety and how to improve the response in case of critical events. Three of the most important models that take into consideration the possibilities and opportunities of dealing and coping with a risk and disaster are discussed here.

The first is named the Pressure and Release Model. According to Wisner et al. (2004), this model "shows in diagrammatic terms how the causes of vulnerability can be traced back from unsafe conditions, through economic and social (dynamic) pressures, to underlying root causes. . . . We can also describe this as a pathway, 'progression of vulnerability' or 'chain of causation,'" This model was useful when it first was elaborated, but it seems to be too static and lacks the coordinates of complexity, simultaneity, and dynamicity.

Instead, another model seems to take into consideration all these aspects. The Access Model "picks up the state of 'normal life' and explains how people earn a livelihood with differential access to material, social and political resources" (Wisner et al. 2004).

The third model is connected with what has been defined as "sustainable livelihood" by Chambers and Conway (1992). It has four types of capital similar to the Access Model (Wisner et al. 2004):

- Human capital (skills, knowledge, health and energy)
- Social capital (network, groups, institutions)
- Physical capital (infrastructures, technology and equipment)
- Financial capital (savings, credit)
- Natural capital (natural resources, land, water, fauna and flora)

This topic is a classical sociological issue because of the access to resources of different types; the possibilities and opportunities that are correlated are the basis of many social research studies, as shown by Coleman (1986) and Bourdieu (1983).

The third model was elaborated not for social scientists, but for practical intents. As Nathan (2005) pointed out, "field workers, unsatisfied with usual mitigation methods, proposed a tool called vulnerability and capacity assessment (VCA), but its reappropriation by social scientists is still in its infancy" and again "the first comprehensive attempt to propose a VCA, from Anderson and Woodrow in 1989, proposed a matrix of vulnerabilities and capacities crossed by three categories":

- Physical/material
- Social/organizational
- Motivational/attitudinal

This model seems to be very operative and practical when evaluating vulnerable situations and conditions because its approach is people-centered and controlled by the exposed people themselves. This element takes into consideration one aspect that is important for a sociological reflection on vulnerability in the risks and disasters field (Bankoff 2004): "vulnerability is also about people, their perceptions and knowledge. People's idea about risk and their practices in relation to disasters constitute the sextant and compass with which they measure and chart the landscape of vulnerability."

A sociological approach to social vulnerability within a risk, crisis, and disaster context lies exactly within this suggestion: the perception of people and their feelings, values, and beliefs should be the indicators followed when planning and understanding, in the best way possible, the vulnerable side of human life and modern societies. In particular, attention is focused on this topic and on the interviews with people affected by an earthquake, which is the *voice of vulnerable people* (Voss 2008).

Another important question to take into account is that vulnerability occurs not only in the phase of prevention and preparedness and does not regarding only "preexisting conditions," as per Villagràn de Leon (2004). Vulnerability, as we see later, is a characteristic throughout all the phases of a disaster: mitigation, preparedness, planning, response, and reconstruction.

In fact, I have had the opportunity to explore how vulnerability, in general terms, is present not only before and in the latent phase of a disaster but also during the response and the reconstruction phases, in which the lack of resources, the different methods of access, influenced and oriented the possibility of "normalization" or resilient activities, also in a community close to another, with diverse effects on the social reconstruction dynamics and the opportunity to come back and live again in the same place.

Finally, it is useful to clarify our intention to use the integrative approach presented by Voss (2008) during the analytical phase of this research. *The approach is subtly based on Turner et al. (2003) although it has been significantly modified. In their approach, Turner and colleagues address both the Risk-Hazard-Approach as well as the Social-Vulnerability-Approach. They define vulnerability as the degree to which a system, subsystem, or system component is likely to experience harm due to exposure to a hazard, either a perturbation or stress/stressor (2003).* The integrative approach seems to be the most useful in the context of social studies on vulnerability, risk, and disaster. This sociological approach takes into account this suggestion, based on the definition of social space and social milieu relationships elaborated by Schultz (1972).

2.5 Risk and Resilience: Toward a Relational Approach of Risk

In the previous paragraphs I presented some core concepts of the sociological framework of crisis, disaster, risk, and resilience (Bohle 2008). In this brief proposal of the relationship between the concepts of risk and resilience, there are some sociological assumptions that need to be considered.

- Risk can be identified as a concept defined by a social process of reality construction (Berger and Luckmann 1966). In particular, it seems interesting to focus attention on the primary and secondary socialization processes and their influence on the perception of risk and the transgenerational dynamics among members of the same family.
- Symbolic interactionism (Mead 1934) based on the consideration of the importance of social interaction and its symbolic identification among people, institutions, and general social organizations.
- Social milieu relationships (Schultz 1972) that focus attention on the relationships between human actions and the physical and social context in which they take place.

Starting our proposal with the consideration of risk as a concept constituted by a social and communicative process (Lombardi 2005), it is important to point out some crucial aspects related to the concept of risk.

- In our complex society risk should be represented as a social process in terms of communication practices (Lombardi 2005), social interaction, social representations, social construction, sense and meaning making, and their related cultural aspects.
- Although this first implication is socially oriented, risk should also be understood in terms of natural and technical features typical of a stressor or agent that can cause a crisis or disaster situation.

Taking into account the historical evolution of the concept of risk and considering all elements present in its definition, we propose another theorization. In a graphical language, without mathematical or measuring expectations, it can be written as follows:

$$R = \left([P \times I] \times [V \times R]^{n} \right)$$

where P is probability and I is intensity – two features of the stressor itself – and V is vulnerability and R is resilience, which are typical features of victims, systems, organizations, and social structures. In this theorization model, risk results from the product of these four factors combined in different ways.

This logic allows us to implement the conceptualization of vulnerability and resilience in a different way than previous theorizations. As mentioned earlier, they are not opposites; instead they are correlated, showing the features of systems or victims potentially at risk.

It should also be considered that this risk representation needs a time specification: the product of vulnerability and resilience can be repeated N times because of the characteristics of the specific vulnerability and resilience of the systems, organizations, social groups, and individuals at risk. Specifically, the final product will be repeated whenever that the features of a single product changes.

According to this perspective, we are able to discuss the diverse components of risk and, in particular, we can consider operative, natural, and technical features of the risk itself. At the same time we take into account the other side of risk constituted by the human, individual, social, and relational aspects of risk. For instance, when a chemical risk occurs, people involved in the decisional process of risk, such as experts, public administrators, and public relation officers, must consider different dimensions of the risk itself, which are not only based on technical assumptions but also involve cultural and social aspects of the specific risk. This seems to be an important turning point because it highlights fundamental issues in risk analysis and risk communication, such as the possibility of:

- exploring and finding the vulnerable and resilient elements present in a society, community, organization, individual, or social group;
- working on the specific dimensions of resilience, as a process, in the context of social systems, organizations, and social groups;
- thinking about the application of a different decisional pattern within the institutions and organizations responsible for risk communication and crisis management;
- understanding the level of risk exposure related to elements and dimensions of resilience better; and
- taking into account all the different perceptions in the context of risk dynamics.

Specific attention should be paid to a diverse model of risk analysis and risk communication based on the graphical representation above. The model considers the framework within which the cultural and social dynamics of risk take place. It is elaborated starting with the analysis of the relationships between the single components, their networks, and interconnections.

It is necessary to specify that this is not a linear vision wherein an element or feature of vulnerability dovetails with an element or feature of resilience in a deterministic approach. It is a dynamic process within which resilient aspects should be considered when referring to the general process of risk. According to this perspective, it is not only a fundamental question of reducing risk to improve resilience: the latter aspect becomes s specific part of risk itself, and it is assumed that resilience can be a component of risk as well as vulnerability.

What must be understood is that this theoretical reflection does not claim to measure all aspects of vulnerability and resilience. There is a part of these two processes that inevitably is latent and unknown, and this part is the final risk that can occur.

In particular, this hypothesis is based on the belief that a part of specific vulnerability and resilience can be known through the specific analysis of technical and operative components of risk and the perceptions of and communication among the people or the systems potentially at risk. Specifically, in a context of risk communication, resilient aspects can be represented by the following elements:

- Trust relationships between all members involved in a risk situation or crisis management
- Trust relationships between mass media and public and institutional authorities responsible for a crisis and emergency response
- Consideration of cultural and social dynamics involved in the construction of risk perception
- Consideration of transgenerational perception of risk and its importance for the population potentially at risk, for instance, regarding natural risk such as earthquakes, floods, and hurricanes
- Resilient relationships, characterized by collaborative and participative patterns, should be developed in the preventive and latent phases of a possible disaster because they could be directly activated if a disaster occurs

All these aspects need to be studied and considered more to comprehend better the possibility of resilience process within our societies. Understanding resilience as a component of risk itself allows us to improve the possibility of risk awareness, focusing attention on the cultural and social meaning of risk as a shared practice among communities that are potentially at risk.

Chapter 3
What Is Resilience? The State of the Art

Chapter 3 presents the definition of the concept of resilience and its evolution during the past four decades. Resilience is a context-sensitive concept, and for this reason its definition is related to the conceptual, cultural, and operative framework of application. Different types of resilience have been identified: ecological, environmental, institutional, infrastructural, organizational, economic, social, community, familial, and individual. Specifically, professional resilience was proposed for civil protection volunteers. In general, even if the type of resilience differs depending on the context of presentation, resilience has been defined as the capacity, ability, or competence to cope with stress, a crisis, or a disaster and bounce back to the preexisting conditions of life.

In the past 20 years, resilience assumed importance within the context of the sociology of disaster, crisis and disaster management, and disaster planning, resulting in resilience being defined from a sociological perspective and a sociological relational approach. This theorization allows resilience to be reconsidered, specifically its features and the disaster planning patterns that come from the combination of the resilient individual and social actions, social relationships, and interactions.

3.1 Introduction

The main topics defining our contemporary societies and its hazards, risks, crises, and disasters were described earlier. It would incorrect to identify our society as the only, or the first in human history, to have been afflicted with risks, crises, disasters. What has changed in our society is the enhancement of new types of risks and disasters, not their presence in the world.

According to this consideration, all people in past eras were, in some way, resilient. Think of past wars and, unfortunately, the terrible experience of the Holocaust, genocides, and other horrible expressions of violent power. An interesting presentation of this issue is the story collection by Jean Pierre Guèno (2002) telling of

B. Lucini, *Disaster Resilience from a Sociological Perspective*, Humanitarian Solutions in the 21st Century, DOI 10.1007/978-3-319-04738-6_3,

French children and their lives during World War II. This touching book demonstrates the importance of hope and resistance when facing the adversities of life.

What is well represented here is the strength and emotions used as active resources to overcome a disaster and loss (Holling and Gunderson 2002). The theoretical and methodological needs of this research were the definition of resilience from a sociological perspective and the original contribution that this discipline can give to the sociologic resilience process in the context of disasters, whether they be natural or technological as well as those caused by human action.

Resilience is not a human or social concept. Instead it is derived from the physical field and means the capacity and the degree to which a metal can resist damage and return to its original state (Cyrulnik and Malaguti 2005). Introducing this concept and its uses in the field of human and social science is not a simple issue; because of its multidimensional characteristics and the variety of aspects involved in it, resilience can be difficult to define (Cyrulnik and Malaguti 2005) in a satisfactory way. Norris et al. (2008) argued that, "when applied to people and their environment, resilience is fundamentally a metaphor" because of the multidimensional features of resilience itself. As Mayunga (2007) pointed out, "conceptualizing resilience in this way may not be desirable because it does not add much to our understanding. The abundance of definitions of disaster resilience and the fact that this concept is shared by many disciplines makes it difficult to have a common definition. Therefore, it is important to set a working definition that will form a basis for discussion."

Furthermore, Shalev and Errera (2008) argued "that resilience might mean different things to different people at different times, that there are many ways to be resilient, and that the main generic attribute of resilience is a sufficient level of stability and regularity under adversity." They also cited that resilience, according to Layne et al. (2007), "should be reserved for conditions in which there is an initial deflection of the relevant outcome measure." Aguirre (2006) has tried to conceptualize resilience, defining it

> as a multi-dimensional and never ending process that incorporates a host of factors, including:
>
> - Past experiences, imagination, creativity or improvisation (and even luck!)
> - Ability to "bounce back" and continue to function
> - Ability to cope with and recover from the impact of the hazard event
> - A system's capability to effectively absorb, respond, and recover from an internally or externally induced set of extraordinary demands
> - Development of a collective and shared vision of dangers and what to do about them; allows for the constant monitoring of threatening contextual conditions
> - Incorporates both an awareness of potential hazards and their physical, biological, psychological, social, and cultural demands, and the taking of action in anticipation of these demands to minimize their effects
> - Requires a paradigm shift to a more holistic, integrated, and collective approach aimed at enhancing safety and security
> - Resiliency is a function of raising awareness, and conscious planning and training
> - Building resiliency is about capacity building and generating adaptability
> - Understanding resilience in the context of vulnerability: must focus on a vulnerability-resiliency paradigm

Resilience has been in a "golden period" in the past few years, especially in psychological and psychoanalytical disciplines, even if is quite difficult find a systematic approach from a sociological perspective. The challenge of this research is to introduce the definitions, uses, and meanings in human and social disciplines that are important to highlighting the theoretical aspects of a possible sociological proposal of resilience processes and dynamics in disaster contexts, with specific reference to natural disasters and the three Italian earthquakes taken into consideration as the research fieldwork.

The first systematic literature review about resilience was presented by Plodinec (2009). His proposal started with the consideration of the importance of studies in the resilience field related to disasters since the 1980s "and was related to the concept of being able to absorb and recover from a hazardous event. Since that time, hybrid definitions have arisen that combine the engineering with the ecological, or the ecological with the behavioural." As noted by other authors, such as Malaguti (2005), it is difficult to find only one way to define the concept of resilience. One interesting classification of disaster resilience is presented by Mayunga (2007):

> For instance, most authors use the term capacity/ability to define the concept of disaster resilience and confine the concept to people, a group of people, a community, or a society. This generally means that, there is an agreement among researchers that the notion of disaster resilience should be associated with the capacity/ability of people, a group of people, a community or a society to cope with disasters. Worth noting also is the wide usage of the term recovery in the definitions. Most authors define the concept of disaster resilience in terms of the speed or how quickly people, a group of people, a community or a society can recover from the disaster impacts.

In general terms, Tierney (2003a, b) identifies four aspects of resilience, according to the fact that

> both the physical and the social aspects of resilience can be conceptualized as consisting of the following properties:
>
> 1. *Robustness*: the ability of elements, systems, and other *units* of analysis to withstand stresses and demands without suffering damage, degradation or loss of function
> 2. *Redundancy*: the extent to which elements, systems, or other units of analysis exist that meet functional requirements in the event of disruption, degradation, or *loss* of functionality of primary systems
> 3. *Resourcefulness*: the capacity to identify problems, establish priorities, and mobilize resources to avoid or cope with damage or disruption; the ability to apply human and material resources to meet priorities and achieve goals
> 4. *Rapidity*: the capacity to meet priorities and achieve goals in a timely manner.

Operative factors contribute to our understanding of vulnerability and resilience (see Cutter et al. 2008):

- Access to resources and political power
- Social capital and social networks
- Beliefs, cultures, and customs
- Socioeconomic and demographic characteristics
- Special needs population (elderly, chronically ill, etc.)
- Type, construction materials, and age of buildings
- Type and density of infrastructure and lifelines

Cited in Voss (2010), Carpenter et al. (2001), propose four empiric indicators concerning the capacity to adapt as a shape of resilience:

- Institutional indicators
- Economic indicators
- Social indicators
- Biological indicators

We will see that this typology of indicators can be correlated with the level of resilience present and its characteristics at the institutional, economic, political, social, and spatial level; "space" is meant as a social and sharing place within which the social relationships typical of humans are present.

It is interesting to present different perspectives about resilience (Kendra and Wachtendorf 2003; Norris et al. 2009; UNISDR, WMO 2012), their definitions (Nixon and Jaswal 2010), and their methodological implications (Kuhlicke 2010) using the above-mentioned classification and then move on to an introduction of theoretical reflections on resilience from human and social approaches. For a logical presentation, the first point presented is resilience using a physical and ecological approach; then institutional, economic, infrastructural, and organizational resilience in a macro context referring to the sociology tradition are considered. Next is the definition of two perspectives of resilience – meso and central level resilience and social, community, and family resilience – which is the core element of this theoretical background and the basis of the next sociological proposal. Finally, the opposite of the macro level – the micro level, comprising individual and personal resilience – is discussed.

Although I am conscious that this is not a historical presentation, I prefer to follow the sociological logic and offer this kind of perspective, which is more useful for the operative analysis about the three Italian earthquakes. The presentation here shows various dimensions of resilience according to their definitions and considering the main features of resilience, such as context sensitivity.

3.2 Resilience by a Physical, Ecological, and Ecosystem Approach

Following the work done by Plodinec (2009), it is possible to argue that resilience has different approaches correlated to the different domains used to explicate resilience in different fieldworks. The first is a physical domain, and it is represented by the following definitions:

- The ability to store strain energy and deflect elastically under a load without breaking or being deformed (Gordon 1978)
- The ability of systems to resist external influences and return to a well-defined state of equilibrium (Pimm 1991, cited in Lorenz 2010)
- Physical: the speed with which a system returns to equilibrium after displacement, irrespective of how many oscillations are required (Bodin and Wiman 2004)

The second is an ecological system domain, which has been defined by diverse authors as follows:

- The persistence of relationships within a system; a measure of the ability of systems to absorb changes of state variables, driving variables, and parameters and still persist (Holling 1973)
- Buffer capacity, or the ability of a system to absorb perturbation, or the magnitude of disturbance that can be absorbed before a system changes its structure (Holling et al. 1995)
- The ability to persist through future disturbances (Abel and Langston 2001)
- Positive adaptation in response to adversity; it is not the absence of vulnerability, not an inherent characteristic, and not static (Waller 2001)
- The transition probability between states as a function of the consumption and production activities of decision makers (Brock et al. 2002)
- The ability of a system that has undergone stress to recover and return to its original state; more precisely, (1) the amount of disturbance a system can absorb and still remain within the same state or domain of attraction, and (2) the degree to which the system is capable of self-organization (Klein, Nicholls and Thomalla 2003)
- The amount of change or disruption that is required to transform the maintenance of a system from one set of mutually reinforcing processes and structures to a different set of processes and structures (Anderies, Janssen and Ostrom 2004)
- Maintenance of natural capital (as the basis for social systems' functioning) in the long run (Ott and Doering 2004)
- The capacity of a system to absorb disturbance and reorganize while undergoing change so as to still retain essentially the same function, structure, identity, and feedbacks (Walker et al. 2004)
- The capacity of linked social-ecological systems to absorb recurrent disturbances... so as to retain essential structures, functions, and feedbacks (Adgeret et al. 2005)
- The ability by an individual, group, or organization to continue its existence (or remain more or less stable) in the face of some sort of surprise .... Resilience is found in systems that are highly adaptable (not locked into specific strategies) and have diverse resources (Longstaff 2005)
- The capacity of a system to absorb disturbance and reorganize while undergoing change so as to still retain essentially the same function, structure, and feedbacks – and therefore the same identity (Resilience Alliance 2006)
- The capacity of a system to tolerate disturbance without collapsing into a qualitatively different state that is controlled by a different set of processes (Resilience Alliance 2009)
- The ability of communities to withstand external shocks to their social infrastructure (Adger 2000) (the domain here is a little different and refers to ecological and social systems)
- The ability to persist (i.e. to absorb shocks and stresses and still maintain the functioning of society and the integrity of ecological systems) and the ability to adapt to change, unforeseen circumstances, and risks (Adger 2003) (the domain here is a little different and is related to ecological and social systems)

Within this approach, resilience is understood through some useful indicators whenever present in the definitions:

- Resilience as ability or capacity; as we will see later, these aspects are present within almost all definitions of resilience from another perspectives. This consideration is also useful to underline the question about "resilience of" something and "resilience to something," as pointed out by Carpenter et al. (2001) cited in Voss 2010). This is a crucial and core question to analyze and try to answer because of its operative implications for future indicators of resilience practices and in the field of training for the population, volunteers, and civil protection officers.
- The presence of a system, not only considered in an "ecological or social" context, where critical events such as disasters or crises take place, but also as a whole set of relationships and interconnections between the system itself and the people living in it
- Shocks, stresses, disturbance, adversity, perturbation, displacement: I am referring here to the characteristics of crisis and emergency definition (see Chap. 2)
- Adaptation, coping, and reorganization practices

All these elements highlight the importance of ecological system perspectives on resilience because of their deep connection with the social system and the ecological social system (Adger 2000). The theoretical link between the ecological and the social systems allows us to point out the sociological reflection by Schutz (1974 ed. 1932) and the introduction of his "social relational milieu." In fact, ecological resilience, or ecosystem resilience, introduces the importance of space and place in terms of physical and spatial as well as social and relational resilience within a sociological understanding. In these terms, the system is the whole of infrastructures, places, and spaces where the social relationships are taking place both physically and symbolically.

It is also important to remember that this vision seems to be based on the assumption of linear feedback, which does not seem useful when referring to complex social systems. Furthermore, "resilience as a system property is not just a determinant of fluctuation beyond balanced states but rather decisive for the persistence of the system or its capacity for absorption in cases of disturbances" (Lorenz 2010).

The next step in this fieldwork is to comprehend the evolutional process represented by the "interacting social and ecological system . . . conceptualized under the terms human-environment systems" (Turner et al. 2003), "socio-ecological systems" (Gallopìn 2006), and "social-ecological systems" (Berkes et al. 1995, (cited in Lorenz 2010). This approach required consideration of references to our contemporary societies and their characteristics of risk and uncertainty. An important example of the theoretical model according to human-ecological and social perspectives was elaborated by Bronfenbrenner in the U.S.A. and by Tousignant and Sioui (2009), in Canada.

This model has been presented by Malaguti (2005). In particular, she points out that the assumption of social ecology is based on the postulate that development is the result of the integration among different levels of systems (regarding, in this context, children):

- Microsystem: the family
- Exosystem: the community
- Macrosystem: culture and society

The first level focuses on the capacities and abilities that families, as social units, have to face a crisis, disaster, or life perturbation. In the next section, particular attention is given to the family resilience paradigm theorized by Walsh (2006) and the important implications connected with my research fieldwork. The second level is represented by the community and the role of social place in a coping capacity and a better way of adapting to life difficulties.

3.3 Environmental Resilience

Environmental resilience, as well as ecological resilience, has an important role within the theoretical and methodological frameworks of the sociology of disaster and disaster planning. We will see that the preexisting conditions of the environment influence the crisis response, displacement, and recovery phases of the disaster process.

In general, environmental resilience was understood as a related concept of ecological resilience but with more attention on the environmental structure and its sustainability (Brand and Jax 2007). This dimension of resilience is particularly important in the displacement and recovery phases of disaster planning and management because of the practical assumptions necessary to relocate disaster victims and cope with the physical impact of the stressor and its features. Specifically, environmental resilience is directly related to the metaphoric and cultural meaning of the sense of community, sense of place, and place attachment (Low and Airman 1992). For this reason, ecological and social resilience are understood as related concepts (Adger 2000). Considering environmental resilience and its latent or present dimensions before a crisis or disaster, we should be aware of the peculiar characteristics of our physical living place and its influence within the social disaster process.

3.4 Institutional Resilience

Another typical dimension of resilience is its involvement within organizational structures and systems and its support in terms of business continuity and guaranteeing the well-being of the whole social system. For this reason, talking about organizational resilience is a better way to introduce and understand the other side of resilience from the macrosystem point of view.

Institutional resilience has been defined by Abesamis et al. (2006) as "formal and informal rules or regulations, that are in force to secure the right of resource exclusion and extraction." Smith (2009) underlines institutional resilience as a "dimension of resilience that is less studied or understood. . . . Specifically, institutional resilience can be comprehended according to four principal themes":

1. Capacity building
2. Self-reliance
3. Accountability
4. Empowerment

The institutional dimension of resilience is a recent argument, and the literature in this field is not well developed; however, what is interesting for this research is the connection between institutional resilience and the civil protection system. The attention on institutional resilience seems to be basilar for the question of security and safety in our era and within the framework of international cooperation actions and programs.

3.5 Economic Resilience

Economic dimensions of resilience can be introduced according to the perspective presented by Rose (2007) as cited by Plodinec (2009), defining economic resilience as:

- Static: "ability of a system to maintain function when shocked (efficient use of remaining resources at a given point in time)"
- Dynamic: "speed of a system to recover from a shock (efficient use of resources over time for investment in repair and reconstruction)"

This conceptual framework is based on the theorization done by Rose (2007) and his mathematical definition of economic resilience as direct economic resilience (DER):

$$\text{DER} = \%\Delta DY\,m - \%\Delta DY \,/\, \%\Delta DY\,m$$

where $\%\Delta DY\,m$ is the maximum percentage change in direct output, $\%\Delta DY$ is the estimated percentage change in direct output, and *DER* is the percentage avoidance of a maximum disruption to a given shock. Considering this perspective in our contemporary time of crisis, it could have interesting implications within financial markets and its influence on the daily life of people.

3.6 Infrastructural Resilience

From a macro level perspective, infrastructural resilience is the last dimension. It is a fundamental macro dimension of resilience, correlated to institutions and organizations, which fit in because some aspects of one are common to the others and have methodological and operative implications within planning activities. Specifically, McDaniels (2009) identified the elements of infrastructural resilience: "cross-sectorial planning for infrastructure resilience faces at least three notable challenges," which are "incomplete incentives, partial information and few opportunities for learning." Attention is focused on the role of the information and communication process as the better way to enhance or maintain the infrastructural resilience when a critical event occurs. Infrastructural resilience is strongly related to business continuity – the stability of a system is based on it and the ability to cope or deal with a crisis and disaster and respond adequately to the needs of the system and the population.

3.7 Organizational Resilience

Deeply connected with the discourse on institutional resilience is the question of the resilient organization and its features. There are differences in the methods, components, and types of organization, including the identity of the members, tasks, competencies, aim, objectives, norms, and sense of belonging in the organization. An interesting classification of a disaster resilient organization, taking into account the resilience hierarchy, is articulated by Eisner (2009):

- Individual resilience
- Internal organization resilience
- Peer organization resilience
- Resilience of cross-sector collaboration
- Resilience of integration with local government through pre-event, response, recovery

All these dimensions of a resilient organization should come round to a "resilient standard" (Eisner 2009), including a "defined strategic disaster mission, hazard assessment, facility resilience, disaster operations plans, response, ops, coop, recovery, intra- and inter-sector support agreements, donations [and] volunteer management, training, exercises [and] continuous improvement, disaster education [and] communication, financial [and] reimbursement system." For the general aim of this contribution, the element of standard resilience, which seems more interesting, lies in disaster operations plans, volunteer management, disaster education, and communication. This is because of the social aspects of the resilience process and the importance assumed by the volunteer to enhance and better comprehend their role and their possible incorporation before, during, and after a disaster resilience process.

3.8 Social Resilience

Social resilience is one of the crucial elements that is present in this sociological proposal for a definition of disaster resilience. It seems useful to note that social resilience from a sociological perspective is quite different from the definition of it by Sapirstein (2006), who focused attention on his own model of resilience, which comprised the following elements: redundancy through overlapping social networks, strengthening response capacities, supporting self-organization, fostering learning and education, and encouraging adaptation.

According to a general view, social resilience, instead, can be defined as the capacity of people in group (formal and informal) to face up to a disaster during the emergency and reconstruction time, starting from collective and individual resources made available for all people involved and with needs to be satisfied through altruistic behavior and shared social relationships. This is a conceptual presentation and focuses on the importance of better understanding the types of capacities and resources already present in a community or society that would be stricken by a disaster. Other definitions of social resilience highlight different characteristics and elements.

1. The presence of two types of social resilience by Kofinas (2003):
    - A social system's capacity to facilitate human efforts to deduce the trends of change, reduce vulnerabilities, and facilitate adaptation
    - The capacity of a (social-ecological system) to sustain preferred modes of economic activity
2. The ability of communities to withstand external shocks to their social infrastructures (Adger 2000)
3. The ability of social units to mitigate hazards, contain the effects of disasters when they occur, and carry out recovery activities in ways that minimize social disruption and mitigate the effects of future earthquakes (Bruneau et al. 2003)

We must recognize that social resilience definitions often are related to the ecological context within which a disaster takes place. An interesting point of view is represented by Lorenz (2010), who, after considering the adaptive capacity and coping capacity at a structural and systemic level, presents participative capacity (Voss 2010) as "the measure of the ability to self-organize and use adaptive and coping capacity."

3.9 Community Resilience

Another perspective presented in the analysis and literature review of resilience definitions by Plodinec (2009) takes into account the community context (Bauman 2001). Declinations about the definitions of resilience include the following:

- The capacity to adapt existing resources and skills to new systems and operating conditions (Comfort 1999)

- (The ability to) withstand an extreme event without suffering devastating losses, damage, diminished productivity, or quality of life without a large amount of assistance from outside the community (Mileti 1999)
- A sustainable network of physical systems and human communities, capable of managing extreme events; during a disaster both must be able to survive and function under extreme stress (Godschalk 2003)
- A system's capacity to absorb and recover from the occurrence of a hazardous event; reflective of a society's ability to cope and to continue to cope in the future (Timmerman 1981)
- The capacity to cope with unanticipated dangers after they have become manifest; learning to bounce back (Wildavsky 1991)
- The ability to recover from or adjust easily to misfortune or sustained life stress (Brown and Kulig 1996)
- The process through which mediating structures (schools, peer groups, family) and activity settings moderate the impact of oppressive systems (Sonn and Fisher 1998)
- The capability to bounce back and to use physical and economic resources effectively to aid recovery following exposure to hazards (Paton and Johnston 2001)
- Intentional action to enhance the personal and collective capacity of its citizens and institutions to respond to, and influence the course of, social and economic change (Center for Community Enterprise 2000)
- The ability to respond to crises in ways that strengthen community bonds, resources, and the community's capacity to cope (Chenoweth and Stehlik 2001)
- The ability of individuals and communities to deal with a state of continuous long-term stress; the ability to find unknown inner strengths and resources in order to cope effectively; the measure of adaptation and flexibility (Ganor and Ben-Lavy 2003)
- Community resilience consists of (1) the amount of change a system can undergo and still retain essentially the same structure, function, identity, and feedbacks on function and structure, (2) the degree to which a system is capable of self-organization (and reorganization after a disturbance), and (3) the degree to which a system expresses capacity for learning and adaptation (Quinlan 2003)
- The development of material, physical, socio-political, socio-cultural, and psychological resources that promote safety of residents and buffer adversity (Ahmed et al. 2004)
- An individual's sense of the ability of their own community to deal successfully with the on-going political violence (Kimhi and Shamai 2004)
- A community's capacities, skills, and knowledge that allow it to participate fully in recovery from disasters (Coles and Buckle 2004)
- The capability of a system to maintain its function and structure in the face of internal and external change and to degrade gracefully when it must (Allenby and Fink 2005)
- The return or recovery time of a social-ecological system, determined by (1) that system's capacity for renewal in a dynamic environment and (2) people's ability to learn and change (which, in turn, is partially determined by the institutional context for knowledge sharing, learning, and management, and partially by the social capital among people) (Gunderson and Folke 2005)

- The ability of community members to take meaningful, deliberate, collective action to remedy the impact of a problem, including the ability to interpret the environment, intervene, and move on (Pfefferbaum et al. 2005)
- The capacity of a system, community, or society potentially exposed to hazards to adapt, by resisting or changing, in order to reach and maintain an acceptable level of functioning and structure. This definition is based on the community and society approach by the Subcommittee on Disaster Reduction (2005)
- The capacity of a system, community, or society potentially exposed to hazards to adapt, by resisting or changing, in order to reach and maintain an acceptable level of functioning and structure (UN/ISDR 2005)
- The ability of the system to withstand either market or environmental shocks without losing the capacity to allocate resources efficiently (Perrings 2006)
- The capability to retain similar structures and functioning after disturbances for continuous development (Liu et al. 2007)
- A process linking a set of adaptive capacities to a positive trajectory of functioning and adaptation after a disturbance (Norris et al. 2008). This definition represents an approach of community and individual resilience

Fundamental studies of resilient communities has been done by Garbarino et al. (1992), specifically the slums of Chicago, and he focuses his attention on some useful indicators for possible resilient communities (as cited in Malaguti 2005):

- The presence of deep and rich formal and informal relationships
- Social and educational services
- Cultural proposals
- Equilibrium between man and nature

What emerged from all of this research is that "the more the adversity affects the intimate sphere and creates isolation, the more difficult it is for the group to develop a community resilience" (Malaguti 2005).[1]

The last level is the macrosystem, and it is represented by the cultural and social context within which a person grows up. In this perspective, the culture assumes a major importance in determining the possibility of being resilient during life adversity or a trauma. As Choler et al. (1995) has elaborated, resilience is also a fact of culture, and what is resilient in Western society will not be resilient in other, different cultures. According to previous studies, this is possible starting with the assumption that each person and group has a specific way of facing grief, loss, and suffering.

What is important as a theoretical concept in presentation, and as analytical tools (Bollin 2003) for some aspects of resilience during the three Italian earthquakes (Bonanno et al. 2002, 2010), is the collective sense-making process made possible by a shared resilience experience (Paton et al. 2001a, b; Pfefferbaum et al. 2005) and the consideration of a sense of belonging and collective identity. As cited in Paton and Johnston (2001), Tobin (1999) described a composite model of resilience concerning psychological precursors of resilience and defined resilience from a

[1] Malaguti (2005): *Più l'avversità tocca la sfera intima e crea isolamento, più sarà difficile per il gruppo sviluppare una resilienza comune.*

social and psychological perspective. "A function of the operation of personal characteristics, the ability to impose a sense of coherence and meaning on atypical and adverse experiences, and the existence of community practices (e.g. supportive social network) which mitigate adverse consequences and maximise potential for recovery and growth" (Violanti et al. 2000).

Some variables are presented to explain better the validity of this theoretical framework (Paton and Johnston 2001):

- Sense of community: "also provides insight into the degree of community fragmentation and, consequently, the level of support likely to exist for collective intervention or mitigation strategies"
- Coping style
- Self-efficacy
- Social support

Other variables useful in understanding the process of community resilience and its empowerment strategies were proposed by Kieffer (1984) and Paton and Bishop (1996), cited in Paton and Johnston (2001). These include:

- Community participation
- Enhancing perceived control
- Facilitating community identification of problems
- Developing strategies to solve or contain problems in ways consistent with the needs, systems and values of a specific community

Again, the same authors list empowerment strategies and preventive planning results based on:

- Identification of a community change agent
- The involvement of community members, providing mutual support (contributing to the development of a sense of community and social support)
- Opportunities to lobby social and political agencies (contributing to the development of efficacy and problem-focused coping)

This theoretical proposal underlines the deep need for a community to be the object of empowerment practices to respond better to a natural, technological, or terrorist crisis or disaster without the need for the agent of their origin. This theoretical approach seems really useful for the analysis of interviews with the populations in each earthquake in later chapter. In fact, the authors highlight the central questions for community resilience and provide methodological instruments to identify it. They also provide operative tools to be applied in the crisis and disaster planning, in spite of the authors themselves considering their proposal as a starting point in this field of study.

Tobin and Whiteford (2002) proposed other variables for resilience studies within their new conceptual model for resilience.

The elements of three separate models have been adapted here to demonstrate how resilient communities might be created.

- The mitigation model proposed by Waugh (1996) with the elements of: theories and goals, capable agencies, leadership and politics, constituency support, long term commitment
- The recovery model described by Peacock and Ragsdale (1997) identified by: re-accumulation of capital, government policies and relief aid, resource distribution
- A structural cognitive model put forward by Tobin and Montz (1997) composed by: structural changes, as societal changes; situational factors as physical location, age, income, health, educational, gender, social networks; cognitive factors as psychological and attitudinal

They have applied this theoretical framework to natural disasters and specifically to the eruption of Tungurahua and the evacuation of the Faldas in Ecuador in 1999, based on the assumption that health status was used as a proximate variable for community resilience (Tobin and Whiteford 2002). General conclusions were expressed as follows: "The result of this research suggests that community resilience and recovery effects need focus on nascent and early health problems that may signal the potential for greater problems, reducing the ability of community members to help their own areas recover" (Tobin and Whiteford 2002).

In general terms, using the approach and its characteristic elements according to the sociological view is possible if we take into account the interconnection between people; define community and context in physical or social areas; and comprehend that "nobody is resilient by oneself, without exceptions: the family, the residential area, the community, the society, the culture completely interacted" (Malaguti 2005; Brenson-Lazan 2003).[2] When a man or woman adapts him/herself to a context he/she becomes a different man or woman and for this reason he or she has influenced the community in which he/she lives (Mead 1966). In particular, "communities have the potential to function effectively and adapt successfully in the aftermath of disasters" (Norris et al. 2008).

I present here the main considerations of community concepts, its definition, and its application in the field of disaster. Talk about resilience placed attention on the evaluation and implementation of resilience itself as defined through the different attributions we are now discussing. According to Blumenfield and Ursano (2008), if we are referring to disaster community resilience we should take into account eight main factors:

- Connectedness, commitment, and shared value
- Participation
- Structure, roles, and responsibilities
- Resources
- Support and nurturance
- Critical reflection and skill building

[2] Malaguti (2005): *Non si è, senza eccezioni, resilienti da soli: la famiglia, il quartiere, la comunità, la società, la cultura interagiscono completamente.*

- Communication (Pfefferbaum et al. 2004, 2007)
- Disaster prevention and mitigation, preparedness and response

Each factor is present in the context of disaster and resilience. All elements of community resilience are connected with the system of emergency response and recovery (Cutter et al. 2003), prevention, mitigation, and preparedness activities. This theoretical analysis and methodological, operative tools allows me to connect these factors within my research context, represented by the three earthquakes in Italy, and make some interesting considerations in the field of disaster resilience and disaster resilient communities.

At the end of this literature review of the concept of resilience and because of their efforts within methodological and practical fieldworks, Plodinec (2009) and the Community & Regional Resilience Institute define community resilience as “the capability to anticipate risk, limit impact, and bounce back rapidly through survival, adaptability, evolution, and growth in the face of turbulent change.”

3.9.1 How to Build Community Resilience

After the analysis of the main theories and methodological framework (Bogardi 2006) within the argument of resilient communities and disaster, it is interesting to take into account the proposal elaborated by Blumenfield and Ursano (2008) on how to build community resilience for disasters.

1. Create consciousness regarding community resilience
2. Foster community development based on input and engagement
3. Adopt a holistic wellness approach
4. Develop and practice disaster plans

The topic of building community resilience includes thoughts about the definition of therapeutic communities and a community strength hypothesis (Bravo et al. 1990).

Community preparedness (Mathbor 2007) should also be linked to the model of community resilience presented by Ronan and Johnston (2005), called SS4R – Strengthening Systems 4R (Risk Reduction, Readiness, Response and Recovery) prevention model. The model focuses on prevention and participative activities that could be done at a community level to enhance the preparedness of a community at risk.

Another reflection concerns a competent community (Sonn and Fisher 1998) and the constitutive elements such as empowerment and adaptive capacity (Zimmermann 2004). Other models (cited in Prati and Pietrantoni 2009) in the field of community resilience are presented here to understand better how to build a resilient community.

- Bachrach and Zautra (1985) identify three variables: auto efficacy, coping oriented to the problem, and sense of community. All three variables have the task

of involving community members within the prevention and preparedness practices in case of crisis and disaster.
- Breton (2001) emphasizes the importance of social capital and social networks among people, groups, and associations present in a community.
- Clauss-Ehelers and Lope-Levy (2002) proposed consideration for the culture of the community, and they identified three different factors of resilience linked to culture: the priority is represented by familiar need; recognition of the authoritative role of older people within a family, with the role of guide; and relationships considered for their internal and deep value.
- At the same level of culture, another interesting approach was proposed by Abramowitz (2005), who, through his anthropological research, found the crucial role played by narrative practices and collective ritual. We will see how this theoretical framework is useful to an analysis of my fieldwork.

According to this perspective, Prati (2006) listed protective factors, such as social factors, cultural factors, economic factors, and political factors. All of them (and their explanations) are useful and necessary to understand community resilience and its influence in crisis and disaster management.

3.10 Family Resilience

Understanding the implications of family within a resilient process during or after a crisis, disaster, loss, or trauma is also important from a sociological perspective. For this reason, it is interesting to consider one of the most important studies and models of this issue, created by Walsh (2006). Walsh (2008) defines resilience as "the ability to rebound from crisis and overcome life challenges."

Confusion about the resilience process is related to the beliefs that people affected by adversity or a critical event feel and use to survive; these are "naturally" resilient. Survival is not the same as resilience; resilience is an active process that requires the involvement of a person and is based on a change of situation and personal and prosocial attitudes to overcome the difficulties (Wolin and Wolin 1993).

Walsh (2006) identifies a conceptual framework to define and analyze family resilience, following its basilar assumption :

1. Family belief system
2. Organizational patterns
3. Communication processes

Walsh started with the system of familiar beliefs and points out the absolute coherence between this approach and the characteristics of contemporary societies. She identifies four essential aspects:

- Varied family structures
- Changing gender roles
- Growing cultural diversity and socioeconomic disparity
- Varying, expanded family life course

The system of beliefs allows us to focus attention on the changes each family experiences and help families find a sense of continuity and coherence during the difficulties and critical events always present in life (Bateson 1994). This aspect is fundamental when referring to the individual and social representations of adversities and the impact of disasters, stress, and trauma.

A practical consideration must be respect for different cultural meanings used by families and for all "diverse images" of a family and their implications. This process has the aim of becoming aware of the different points of view and the complexity of human experiences (Gergen 1991).The first element to take into consideration is the system of beliefs – defined by Gergen (1991) and Hoffman (1990) – as a social construction evolving into a continuous process upon interaction with others and the wider social context (Walsh 2006).

What is important to note is that, even in a psychological and clinical context, this approach could considered in a sociological field because of the following theoretical and methodological implications:

- The importance attributed to the sharing of symbolic and practical beliefs among all family members and in a community context in general
- The importance of making the suffering and sorrow evident during and after a critical event
- Making sense of the adversity and sharing the critical situations with the support and help of all family members. It has been demonstrated that this process is basilar for family resilience (Antonovsky 1988; Patterson and Garwick 1994)
- Giving a sense of coherence and a narrative structure to the worst experiences of life allows us to maintain and perpetuate our own familial history and community history in general: "meanings and the beliefs are expressed in the narratives we construct together to make sense of our world and our position in it" (Walsh 2006)
- Normalizing and contextualizing the adverse experience
- Comprehending the differences and the characteristics of attributive beliefs and explicative beliefs
- Understanding the importance of religious or other kinds of values used to overcome a crisis or disaster and, maybe, to become resilient or more resilient than before the critical situation
- The role of courage and trust during all the phases of a crisis and disaster and their importance for a resilient response to the critical events of life

All these aspects belonging to the clinical field also connect with the sociological elements present before, during, and after a crisis or disaster. In fact, the beliefs that are typical of a community or a group of people (a family unit as well as other social groups) have a strong role in influencing and orienting the possibility to cope and deal with a critical situation. Many researches in this field have focused attention on this issue and found that the general attitude in the face of a crisis or disaster can interpret the way in which a crisis or a disaster can be managed.

The interpretation of a critical element is fundamentally a sociological issue because of its influence on the political, cultural, economic, and social organizations stricken by a crisis. The elements of trust, hope, and optimism are deeply present in any sociological discussion about social relationships, which constitute the core aspects of social life. In particular, this point is well expressed by the symbolic interactionism and the importance given to social and sharing processes such as communication and interaction.

The second aspect on which Walsh (2006) focused her proposal is organizational structures and models. As she points out, "family organizational patterns are maintained by internal and external norms, influenced by cultural and family belief systems." Walsh presents three key concepts that are important for the understanding of this context: flexibility, connectedness, and social and economic resources. This proposal concerning different organizational and familiar models is important if connected with sociological theory and the useful analysis of frameworks for crisis and disaster management models use to respond better to critical events.

An organizational system, for example, the civil protection system, is based on some basilar principles and norms, even if it has changed a little within its own culture despite recent difficulties, in particular the major participation of citizens and the at-risk population according to evaluations by scientific institutes and central, regional, departments of Italian civil protection. This is just a small step on this issue, and much work must be done to fill the unfair disparity always present in Italy because of geographical, economic, political, and social differences.

The proposal by Walsh (2006) presented briefly here allows us to go deep into the field of family resilience; it tries to explicate family resilience focusing on the sociological aspects of this process, in particular the reciprocal and circular exchanges of help among family members facing a disaster, the symbolic meanings present in all families when identifying a crisis or a disaster and proposing an adequate response to them, and the transgenerational aspects of perceived risks and disaster meaning. The importance of this kind of resilience is the foundation of my analysis of the specific earthquakes in Umbria and Molise, where the fundamental question of family resilience and the need to support and enhance it during all phases of disaster appeared.

3.11 Individual and Psychological Resilience

It is impossible not to mention another important approach to resilience: the individual and psychological one, as Richardson (2002) describes: "research in psychiatry and psychology tends to approach resilience as an individual phenomenon. From the 1970s, psychologists have continued to explore the individual qualities that enable people to deal effectively with adversity. Traits such as self-mastery, self-efficacy, positive outlook, and sense of humour have been isolated as contributing to resilience in the general population."

At the same time Plodinec (2009) identifies the definitions of resilience from an individual point of view:

- the process of, capacity for, or outcome of successful adaptation despite challenging or threatening circumstances (Maste et al. 1990)
- the capacity for successful adaptation, positive functioning, or competence... despite high-risk status, chronic stress, or following prolonged or severe trauma (Egeland et al. 1993)
- good adaptation under extenuating circumstances; a recovery trajectory that returns to baseline functioning following a challenge (Butler et al. 2007)

Other definitions of resilience have been collected by Shalev and Errera (2008), adapted from Layne et al. (2007):

- Pathways to competent adaptation despite exposure to conditions of adversity (Cicchetti 1996)
- The individual's capacity for adapting successfully and functioning competently despite experiencing chronic stress or adversity, or following exposure to prolonged or severe trauma (Cicchetti and Rogosch 1997)
- The possession and sustaining of key resources that prevent or interrupt loss cycles (Hobfoll et al. 2000)
- The ability of adults... who are exposed to potentially disruptive events to maintain relatively stable healthy levels of psychological and physical functioning (Bonanno 2004)

In my fieldwork, resilience has required giving attention to protective factors, for example (Castelli 2011):

- Cognitive abilities
- Positive vision of oneself and one's own life
- Sense of safety
- Positive temperament
- Internal locus of control
- Prosocial personality
- Capacity of regulation and self-control

These factors are individual factors. Instead, many other studies have organized their theoretical proposal around the relationships among people and the relationships among individuals and context (Garmezy 1985; Overstreet et al. 1999; Luthar et al. 2000; Nettles et al. 2000; Masten 2001).

As previously mentioned, resilience is defined, in general terms, as a process to enhance health and quality of life (Malaguti 2005). Gamerzy (1991) points out the importance of adaptation or nonadaptation and the interrelation between the two dynamics. Patterson (2001, 2002a, 2002b) defined resilience as the capacity to function in an adaptive way and become competent in spite of a stressful situation or critical event, and he identifies these situations as the "agent of resilience," that is, the emergent condition of the process of resilience.

Empowerment (Rappaport 1977, cited in Malaguti 2005) "is the process with the aim of the acquisition of the power that is the enhancement of the capacities of singles and groups in the active control of their lives." Zimmerman (1999, cited in Malaguti 2005) defined empowerment as a "multilevel concept at individual (psychological), organizational, social or communitarian" level. All these aspects require a high level of personal involvement for an individual person living in a critical situation. Control and the possibility of being active in a stressed or critical situation are the basis for the empowerment concept and future resilience process. Within the clinical area of intervention, empowerment is understood to enhance the ability and the capacity of people to use their own resources to improve their personal response to a critical event or situation.

3.12 Professional Resilience as a Proposal

The main contributions to resilience definitions and their theoretical frameworks and operative fieldworks were presented above. Considering the issues of this particular research, exploring resilience through three earthquakes in Italy, it was necessary to figure out the complex interconnection between a sort of "professional resilience" expressed by the work of the civil protection volunteers and emergency volunteers in general and the resilience of the population affected by an earthquake at different levels: individual, communitarian, and social. This also represents the main hypothesis on which the development of this research was based, and, for professional resilience, it was the starting point for some considerations.

First, the collaborative correlation between the civil protection volunteers and the population of earthquake victims has an implicit relationship based on resilience actions. On the one hand the population's actions after the earthquakes could be represented as community or social resilience, on the other hand the civil protection volunteers are the representation of "professional resilience." We could refer to professional resilience as "the proactive and prosocial attitudes oriented to help people affected by disaster in a professional way, and, at the same time, helping colleagues trying to avoid burn out or other diseases among the colleagues themselves." In this context, professional people are trained to be resilient, responding in the best way possible to the needs of the victims or population involved in a crisis or disaster.

Professional resilience also addresses the improved capacity to cope with crises and disasters on the basis of some cultural, social, and human attitudes. For instance, during the past 60–65 years, we have seen the implementation of welfare policies and public interventions to guarantee the basic concrete conditions of life for all people. This new way of thinking about the problem of vulnerable social groups and people with hardships in many contexts of daily life has enhanced the coming of professional helpers such as social workers and psychologists. This approach is sociologically rooted within the Weberian perspectives on the difference between profession and mission and their peculiarities.

Specifically, it is important to discuss the possibility of considering the civil protection volunteering as a voluntary service based on relational help and social support (Kaniasty and Norris 1995, 2004; Kaniasty et al. 1990) to enhance and improve resilience at different levels: individual, community, social. This possible process is referred to as personal resilience belonging to the volunteers at these levels:

- Personal and familial
- Peer-to-peer resilience among all other volunteers
- Between the volunteers and the community in which they live
- Between the volunteers and institutions of the Civil Protection Voluntary Service, such as association and voluntary groups at national, regional, provincial, and local levels

These reflections represent part of the theoretical assumptions (Lin 2002; Penner 2002; Licursi 2010) that explore the civil protection volunteer system and its tasks, competencies, skills, and tools within crisis, emergency, and disaster management. This consideration must take into account some interesting elements of helping relationships during critical events, such as:

- Human trust
- Supportive relationship between the volunteers and the people affected by a crisis and disaster
- The identification and awareness of two kinds of dynamics involving the civil protection volunteers: personal and professional
- Show their own feelings to avoid burnout
- Think about better strategies to fit in with the emergency intervention
- The limits and difficulties of this typical social and personal relationship
- Focus attention on the communication help process, its messages, and channels

Finally, we should consider that professional resilience is not only based on capacities used to avoid burn out. It also is based on the collaborative and organizational patterns that make up the civil protection organizations in which the volunteers are involved. According to these aspects, we can understand the importance of preventive training activities and shared meetings for all volunteers involved in emergency management. In particular, these educational activities allow the possibility of creating a "voluntary subculture" within a voluntary organization that can be proposed in time of crisis and emergency to respond in a coordinated way to disasters that occur.

3.13 Disaster Resilience Definition from a Sociological Perspective

Resilience has many areas of application, dimensions, and indicators (Embrace 2012), but until now, attention within the sociological area of disaster research has focused on many different domains of resilience, and no specific consideration has been presented in connection with sociological theories and approaches (Lucini 2013). For instance, during the last 20 years, many studies and research have been oriented on measuring the level of resilience for each context potentially at risk (Cutter et al. 2010; Embrace 2012).

The various indicators, which were elaborated at different levels and aimed to know and measure the resilience concept, are useful and necessary for operative analyses during all phases of a disaster and for the presence of resilience itself. Based on these assumptions, I propose the following definition of disaster resilience from a sociological perspective; this is not aimed at measuring resilience but instead tries to define it as a fundamental concept within the social science approach.

> Disaster resilience can be identified as a primary and secondary socialization process, constituted by the combination of preexisting individual and social actions, interactions and prosocial attitudes (solidarity, social cohesion, altruism) such as latent or learned behaviours and strategies in a situated context, aimed at coping with critical events and expressed in various patterns of disaster management and response: conflicting, narrative, collaborative, coordinative, supportive and resigned. These patterns can be presented in a mixed way, according to different models of crisis and emergency response elaborated by institutions and communities at risk.
>
> Furthermore, each pattern is present within the identification of various dimensions and their strategies within a multidimensional framework that can be considered in our complex contemporary societies:
>
> - Social dimension and its strategies
> - Cultural dimension and its strategies
> - Organizational, infrastructural, and political dimension and its strategies
> - Economic dimension and its strategies
> - Environmental dimension and its strategies
> - Communicative dimension and its strategies

According to this perspective, disaster resilience is represented by the individual and social actions that result from the interconnection of these structures and strategies. The actions are aimed at coping with and responding to crises or disasters from diverse points of view and are related to the operative indicators presented by the Embrace project (2012).

The theoretical level of the above definition and its interpretation of disaster resilience are influenced by the following sociological theories.

- Symbolic interactionism (Mead 1934) and its attention to social and communicative processes. In cases of crisis and disaster, communication and information (Habermas 1980) are useful activities to enhance our knowledge for preventive planning, preparedness activities, and emergency response.
- Note the importance of social relational milieu as presented by Schutz (1974 ed. 1932), with importance given to the environment, social space, and symbolic place, which should be taken into consideration during the specific phase of disaster: evacuation, displacement and coming back home.
- Different socialization patterns and models are present in each community affected by a critical event, starting with the sociological assumption by Berger and Luckmann (1966), that everything is socially constructed.
- Sense- and meaning-making processes occur according to the cultural framework that characterizes the social systems stricken by critical events.

Furthermore, referring to the previous analytical work done by the experts of the Embrace project (2012), we can identify some operative categories to understand better whether disaster resilience is present and how it is represented in term of features and strategies:

- *Social category*: the presence or absence of trust and community relationships, social capital, solidarity, social cohesion, prosocial attitudes, sharing resources and information, fruitful interaction between different agencies, social and civil participation, stakeholders who can be involved to support and help the network in case of emergency or crisis
- *Cultural category*: the presence or absence of a resilient subculture among social groups with different social and cultural backgrounds and cultural heritage and the interaction among their meaning in terms of crisis, emergency, and disaster situations; possibility to share a common cultural background that creates a cultural and social identity
- *Organizational, infrastructural, and political category*: the presence or absence of collaborative, coordinating, and efficient interactions among diverse institutional and nonprofit agencies that could be involved in the management of a possible crisis or disaster. In particular, the role of political agendas and public policies should be considered to enhance social and community resilience during critical events
- *Economic category*: the presence or absence of material and economic resources that can be used in times of emergency and during the preventive phase to enhance training activities and informational campaigns
- *Environmental category*: the presence or absence of environmental considerations in terms of awareness about the physical context within which we live and the possible risks and vulnerability that it presents for mankind and for itself; place attachment and place identity
- *Communicative category*: the presence or absence of preventive, emergency, and risk communication that would have resilient features in terms of efficacy, dissemination, content of the message, robustness of the communicative channel, and adequacy of the communicative policies

For future methodological applications of this theoretical model in the fieldwork of three earthquakes in Italy, it is necessary to specify that we are referring to the elaboration of operative indicators that can be found within the project Embrace (2012). In particular, I have tried to consider the dimensions of each context and the possibility of finding them related to specific patterns of disaster management and response. That an organized and structured voluntary service such as the Civil Protection Voluntary Service is an important resilient element to cope with critical events also has been assumed.

Chapter 4
Organizational Response to Emergencies: Italian Civil Protection and Civil Defence Service

This chapter describes the evolution of the Italian Civil Protection Service and its theoretical and operative frameworks through the consideration and analysis of laws and decrees that established the actions, skills, roles, and competencies for this fundamental system. In particular, since the end of World War II, the Civil Protection Service was considered the main operative and methodological service in terms of crisis and emergency response: in this period civil protection actions were aimed at response and recovery activities. During the past 60 years there has been a change of perspective, and attention became focused on the peculiarities and communication needs during the prevention, preparedness, and warning phases. The Italian Civil Protection Service also is presented according to the institutional framework of the vertical and horizontal principle of subsidiarity. With regard to this organizational structure, all civil protection activities are related to four contexts of application: local, provincial, regional, and national. A last feature of this system is the presence of civil defense and the fire service within the same organizational framework as the Italian Civil Protection Service.

4.1 Italian Civil Protection Service

In Italy, the National Civil Protection Service has been identified as all structures and activities used by the nation to safeguard the integrity of life, goods, settlements, and the environment from damage or threats caused by natural calamities, catastrophes, and other critical events. The current organizational and systemic complexity of our society means that emergency management has a specific feature that is a peculiar activity of the state: it does not have an exclusive centralized jurisdiction but is a shared issue between the central State, regions, and local administrations; in Italy, this is unusual compared to many other activities.

Laws presented during the Bassanini Reform in 1997 applied the logic of decentralization or devolution. This Reform became effective through Reform V of the

B. Lucini, *Disaster Resilience from a Sociological Perspective*, Humanitarian Solutions in the 21st Century, DOI 10.1007/978-3-319-04738-6_4,

Italian Constitution upon enactment of constitutional law no. 3 (2001). Principles such as the vertical and horizontal subsidiarity have been identified in reference to the decentralization logic. This framework is deeply rooted in the historical and political processes that occurred during those years 1980s–1990s, but it is also connected with the cultural aspect: subsidiarity as well as voluntary service correspond to both cultural indicators and social ones in Italian culture and traditions.

The Civil Protection Service often is identified with the famous statement by Emperor Ottaviano Augusto: "the value of planning diminishes with the complexity of the state of the things." Therefore, more complexity should determine more innovations and developments within emergency management planning, prevention, and preparedness activities.

The Italian National Civil Protection Service is organized according to the plan of prevision, prevention, rescue, and restoration. In the field of prevision, the Service is involved in the study and research of calamitous phenomena, with the support of National Research Institute, to develop specific territorial mapping (made possible through scientific and institutional contributions) of areas at major risk from natural phenomena and man-made disasters and monitoring of areas at high risk for calamitous events. Prevention is constituted by all activities that allow risks connected with calamitous events to be avoided or reduced and make possible informative and training courses for the population at risk. Rescue activity consists of interventions directed toward a primary form of first aid for the civilian population affected by any disaster. Finally, restoration comprises all activities that aim to create a state equilibrium that is typical of the time before critical events.

4.2 The History of the Civil Protection System: From the Unity of Italy to World War II

Natural disasters, disasters caused by human actions, and technological disasters in the industrialization era have always been a source of concern and have been interpreted by both experts and the general population. In particular, the general population has contributed to the creation of myths in an attempt to comprehend natural calamities. It is important to remember that, in the past, attention focused on the causes of a calamitous event.

Regarding the historical period and the specific geographical context of a disaster, each community created a culture of signs and symbols that were useful in allowing the perception of risk and its social construction to be shared by all people within the same community and became typical for that social group. Some examples can be identified in some stories of the *Bible* as well as amazing stories about earthquakes, tsunamis, and dragons within Japanese culture. The interpretation of risk by populations (in particular in Western countries) has been influenced by Catholic culture and Aristotelian philosophy. The Renaissance marked a cultural change in the interpretation of the causes of natural calamities. In fact, in this period threats from the degradation of nature and landscapes led to the first political and economic changes.

More recently, because of the large number of victims affected by some natural disasters, the social/collective imagination of the causes of natural calamities focused on the first systematic and scientific studies using instruments and tools constructed to predict earthquakes and seaquakes.

With contributions from different experts, Italy began a systematization of works based on the major natural calamities that had already afflicted the nation. The history of civil protection in Italy started after the Unity of Italy; before that time, the concept of civil protection seemed confusing and was divided at the local level, resulting in extreme fragmentation and the dispersal of energy and resources. This fragmentation was neither useful nor efficient for an effective response to emergencies that, in the specific historical period, were caused by a natural disaster or war.

To better understand this period, we must take into consideration the incredible changes in Italy on multiple levels: political and institutional, legislative, social, and cultural. The aim was to create unification within the country, not only at territorial and political levels but also involving cultural aspects of life. In the context of the era, this aspect was, perhaps, not voluntary, but a deeper analysis of the situation makes the unification quite visible, and it assumed a fundamental importance in the years following.

In this period of reorganization at all levels of national life, civil protection was treated piecemeal and was utilized only in the periods after the emergency in major situations and in the organization of rescue activities. Nowadays this practice has changed, and the organization of civil protection and, more important, the value of prevention are the subject of many conferences, scientific meetings, studies, research, and discussions. Some interesting activities have been organized for the population to test their basic knowledge of emergency response.

The Messina earthquake in 1925 was the critical event that provoked new reflections on the civil protection system in Italy and determined the starting point for many studies and much research. The first law for civil protection also was enacted in 1925: law no. 473 identifies, for the first time, the Labour Ministry and classifies health officials as members of the civil protection system.

In this period, disasters were seen as being caused by natural phenomena such as earthquakes and floods; warnings to populations at risk were nonexistent, scientific studies about the probability of disasters and the use of technological tools were less diffused, and prevention and preventive activities were accepted with difficulty by major experts.

Law no. 833 (1928) was the first law that tried to systematize the civil protection organization. It specified the public organization and identified the practical steps to be applied during an emergency. In this way, emergency and disaster management law was created systematically, even if the conceptual framework of these activities was to have many modifications during the next historical period.

World War I – which occurred before the period being discussed here – provides a useful indicator about the treatment of civil protection activities in Italy: civil protection occurred after big events with many victims and provided inadequate crisis management. With the coming of World War II, however, the civil defense force played a major role. In particular, the civil defense system assumed a relevant role during these two world wars because of the fundamental need to guarantee the safety of the civilian population and the continuity of political activities within a specific logistical and military framework, especially that involving necessary communication between institutional agencies and the military.

Civil defense actions are specifically linked to the political and military activities of that historical period. In particular the actions of this system include maintaining the safety and integrity of the civilian population and The defending places and infrastructures considered to be vital to the well-being of the nation. Because of this organization and the historical context, only after World War II did it become possible to fully comprehend the role of civil protection activities for the future of a new (postwar) nation.

4.3 From 1970 to 1990

The history of civil protection and its distinction as a fundamental activity guaranteeing the safety and development of a country assumed a major role in the middle of the 1970s, when many dramatic events occurred that focused attention not on the cause of the events but on the best practices for managing a crisis and responding to a disaster. In this period many research programmes were done aiming to gain a better understanding, from a scientific and empirical point of view, of natural hazards and their possible consequences.

A useful and critical analysis of diverse crisis and disaster scenarios has allowed me to indentify some interesting indicators of major catastrophes during this time. One was inadequate attention on the use of technologies to prevent and monitor events and their related risks. A second indicator was inadequate information and training provided to the population during the prevention phase. On one hand, the population itself can impede the work of relief and rescue teams; on the other, they could also be a valid support if there is a feeling of personal safety that permits people to be more aware about what they can or should do in cases of emergency or during a disaster. This consideration also is based on the assumption that the active participation of a population during the relief phase is better for the public authorities, allowing them to create a cognitive framework within which it is possible to influence and orient the best response to an emergency and promote more resilient behavior among the population and the relief teams.

Another event that is formative for the civil protection organization is an industrial accident that occurred in Lombardia, Seveso, in 1976. This event determined a change in the popular conceptions of industrial risk. In fact, before this accident, people believed that security in a chemical firm was an internal feature and that there were no external risks to the environment surrounding a firm or the population close to it. However, this accident made clear a new position in terms of the awareness and safety of the civilian population. After this event in Italy, the first Seveso directive (Legislative Decree no. 334 [1999], directive 96/82/CE) was enacted, with the aim of laying the base for future security features in chemical firms.

The activity of civil protection increased with Law no. 966 (1980)" "Law about the relief and assistance to the population affected by a calamity – civil protection." This was the first step toward the creations of the civil protection service, which was realized in 1992. This law has a peculiar aspect: the definition of natural calamities or catastrophes as "situations arising which can result in serious damage or the threat of serious damage to the safety of people and goods and that, by their nature or extent, must be handled with extraordinary interventions." This law defines the tasks of the Ministry of the Interior, which gives general guidelines during any civil protection issue and in cases of calamity. The minister of the interior assumes the role of director of operations and coordinates public administrations (regions, provinces, municipalities).

Furthermore, an interministry committee of civil protection was assigned the tasks of and economic study and planning, coordination of emergency plans, promotion of studies of government interventions to be adopted during the relief phase and aftermath, and promotion of the collection and dissemination of every piece of information useful for the protection of the civil population. A general civil protection board also was formed, constituting fire control services and an interministry technical commission. Some notes in this law also concern the possibility of future collaboration among regional members and municipalities based on actual needs.

The Ministry of the Interior enables all actions necessary to guarantee the following services in case of a natural calamity or catastrophe: urgent technical interventions and first aid and relief assistance to the population affected by a critical event. The former tasks are those of the National Fire Department, which, in the future, will be the primary operative and technical service within the organization of Italian Civil Protection System. The National Fire Department was founded following Law no. 469 (1961).

Law no. 966 also indicates the way in which the Italian civil protection system will be shaped in the next years and the problematic issues with attributing roles and competencies at institutional, political, and administrative levels.

A complete analysis must also consider the practical regulation of Decree no. 66 (1981). It affirms that civil protection is a primary task of the State. This point is interconnected with the general issues of security and safety, in particular in a globalizing world, and the interpretation of security as a fundamental human right; the State must be able to organize itself for an effective and systematic response that is coherent and functions for the security of the nation and its population.

Civil protection is involved in the following areas:

- Prevention of calamitous events through the identification of their origins and causes
- Preparation and realization of first aid and rescue services
- Preparation and realization of rescue services and assistance services provided to the civilian population affected by a critical event

- Coordination of all actions by public administrations, regions, and territorial and institutional agencies during a critical event

Decree no. 66 also identified all members of the civil protection system: Ministry of the Interior, General Director of Civil Protection and Fire Service, the extraordinary commissioner, the commissioner of the state in the region, the prefect, the regional or interregional inspector of the National Fire Department, and the mayor as state officer. The formal elements of the civil protection organization are the:

- Civil protection interministerial committee
- Technical interministerial committee
- Civil protection regional committees

Another member that should be considered in the future is the so-called COC, the Operative Combined Center (in Italian, the Centro Operativo Combinato), which could be activated along the guidelines of Ministry of the Interior. The COC would direct and civil protection activities, with the following tasks:

- Collect and evaluate any information useful to the Civil Protection System
- If necessary, alert the administrations and agencies that will handle the intervention and rescue tasks
- Receive directives from the major institutions regarding rescue activities and assistance and foster actions within the organization
- Collect all data from the area stricken by the critical event and data regarding resources available for aid, rescue, assistance, and relief; further evaluate them and make all the necessary arrangements
- Balance all the interventions among the different agencies involved
- Collect all claims for materials and equipment necessary for rescue and assistance activities
- Promote all the necessary resources with the aim of restoring all essential services in the area stricken by the disaster

In these circumstances, the prefect assumes the role of controlling and directing the agencies that must manage the crisis. The prefect is in the middle level of administration and territorial institutions, which are tasked with first aid and crisis management. In particular, the prefect can activate two other operative instruments or temporary coordination agencies: the CCS (Centro di coordinamento dei soccorsi, or Rescue Coordination Center) and the COM (Centro operativo misto, or Operative Joint Center).

According to Decree no. 66 (1981), there are some specific and sometimes technical activities that characterize emergency management.

- Rescue and relief of victims, preservation of goods, demolition of buildings, and other urgent technical services
- Temporary recovery of victims and health assistance
- Regulation of communications and traffic flow
- Temporary buildings for public offices

- Preparation for a return to the conditions before the emergency, starting with public administrations
- Recovering, keeping, and managing dead animals

These tasks are realized with the help of Assistance Units of Emergency, which are a necessary resource in any emergency situation.

The second part of this decree focuses on the provincial emergency plan and preparation, the people involved, and simulations as fundamental for prevention activities and first aid assistance centers. The third part of the decree regards the reports of emergencies by public or private agencies and activation and predisposition of the civil defense area. In particular, it focuses on first aid, immediate provision of technical services, and the restoration of infrastructural networks, public transportation, and communication links. Attention also is focused on external aid made possible by donations from other countries and states.

Another law to be considered in this legislative and organization analysis of the Italian Civil Protection System is the President of Ministries Council Decree no. 112/1990, a "Regulation regarding the institution and organization of the Civil Protection Department in the field of Presidency of Council of Ministries." This law is fundamental because it outlines competencies and roles in the field of civil protection. In particular, the Civil Protection Department is appointed the following tasks:

- Promoting and connecting initiatives and structures, including voluntary services, at a central level, that are useful to the National Civil Protection Service
- Collecting and disseminating data regarding the prevision and prevention of emergencies
- Managing relationships between administrations, members, and organizations in Italy as well as in foreign countries that focus attention on the relevant scientific activities of civil protection
- Coordinating national civil protection plans or other related plans covering specific regions "at risk"
- Coordinating the realization of emergency plans and the use of resources, including those of the voluntary services, with the activities of rescue and civil defense services
- Disseminating information and training that can be directed toward a culture of prevention among the population
- Coordinating administrations and organizations interested in interventions of civil protection
- Managing activities linked to the restoration of damaged buildings and realization of emergency public building
- Managing and documenting general affairs
- Identifying and training civil protection voluntary associations and groups
- Managing organizational and instrumental activities useful for the working of the department

At this point I proceed with an explanation of the main law in Italian civil protection legislation, that is, Law no. 225/1992 (Severi 1996), "Institution of the National Civil Protection Service." The general aim of the National Civil Protection Service is to "safeguard the integrity of life, goods, settlements and the environment from damage or from the threat of damage caused by natural calamities, catastrophes or other calamitous events." The law promotes coordination of and collaboration between all administrative agencies at different levels.

Events that are of interest to the National Civil Protection Service include:

- Natural events caused by human activities that can be handled with interventions by local administration through laws
- Natural events caused by human activities that, by their nature and extent, require a coordinated intervention by administrations and agencies
- Natural calamities, catastrophes, or other events that, because of their intensity and extent, require extraordinary means/resources and powers

The law takes into consideration what the civil protection activities should be according to the phases of prevision, prevention, rescue, and restoration. It also defines the direction and the coordination of these activities and the national operative structures that constitute the Service. According to the vertical subsidiarity principle, the competencies are attributed to regions, provinces, and municipalities. Other important members of the National Civil Protection Service are the national groups doing scientific research and that collaborate with the Department for Scientific Studies regarding specific issues as well as voluntary associations, which are a source of different resources for many activities. It is important to note that this is a law specific to the Civil Protection Department because it establishes the competencies of each member and all the structures within the same national service.

Another interesting document used to understand the evolution of civil protection in Italy is the Presidency Ministerial Council Decree no. 429/1998, "Regulation regarding the organization and functioning of the National Commission for Prevision and Prevention of Big Events." This law is deeply connected with the new cognitive and practical context of everyday life. For this reason, risks are now defined as "big" according to their impact in terms of spatial and temporal changes in conditions. The National Commission for Prevision and Prevention of Big Events works within the Civil Protection Department and is proactive in the case of prevision and prevention activities; it uses its own methods for organizing and coordinating specific activities. In particular, this law envisages the scenario of international crisis or terroristic attacks, which are typical of our postmodern societies.

4.4 The New Century

In the 21st century, one important step in the civil protection field is represented by Law no. 401/2001, covering urgent dispositions to guarantee the operative coordination of structure with the aim of civil protection activities. The joint committee comprising members of state, regional, and local administrations has been founded within the Presidency of Council of Ministries. This expresses that civil protection has become a concurring issue between the state, regions, and municipalities.

This change makes two considerations possible. (1) The choice to institute civil protection as a concurring issue among different institutional levels is understandable through national (Italian) and European reforms trying to attribute more power in this field to local administrations. (2) This choice seems to respond to strategic and functional needs in terms of personnel, logistics, and economic resources.

The National Seismic Service, the National Commission for the Prevision and Prevention of Big Events, and the Civil Protection Operative Committee were activated within the Presidency of Council of Ministries. The Civil Protection Operative Committee assures the unitary direction and coordination of emergency activities, establishing the agencies and administration providing rescue activities. The activities of the Civil Protection Department also are defined in this legal framework according to the regional and local context and are based on the emergency plan, interventions, and organizational structure necessary to cope with calamitous events. It is also important to remember the role of coordination played by the prefect concerning the aspects of control and public order.

Within the 21st century, and considering the terrorist attack that occurred in the U.S.A. on September 11, 2001, particular attention has been paid to the implementation of civil defense activities, but here I specify what that means for Italian civil defense. The Presidency of Council of Ministries decree of March 2, 2002, incorporated the Civil Protection Operative Committee within the civil protection system: Its aim is to guarantee the unitary direction and the coordination of emergency activities. In the same law there is a specific section related to its composition and functioning.

Another decree on April 12, 2002, established the constitution of the National Commission for Prevision and Prevention of Big Events. This commission works within the Civil Protection Department and provides scientific support. The law determines the composition, sections, organization, and functioning of this commission. This National Commission is divided into the following categories of risk: seismic, volcanic, hydrogeological, industrial, chemical, nuclear, transport, infrastructural and civil, forest fire, environmental and health, and the defense of cultural heritage from natural risks and risks caused by human actions. What is important to note is the necessity for balance among these sections to overcome the boundaries between them.

An interesting document was one published on September 30, 2002, concerning "The distribution of administrative competencies for civil protection." The introduction of this document is about the normative framework of the Civil Protection Service. Then competencies, roles, and functions of different members are specified, after which the Bassanini Reform is recognized as necessary for emergency management at different levels. The Civil Protection Department has the competencies for technical and operative activities and, according to the regional guidelines, identifies the interventions and the organizational structure necessary to cope with a critical event.

Furthermore, the Civil Protection Department is responsible on three levels.

1. It proposes guidelines, as well as methods for their promotion and coordination, to the president of the council.
2. It is involved in the operative functions of prevision and prevention programs.
3. It highlights attention on the necessary guidelines for operative coordination between private and public administrations and agencies.

The regions are responsible for prevision and prevention activities and urgent interventions during calamities and other necessary missions for recovery and to return balance to that before the crisis. The provinces have competencies for the provincial emergency plan and the realization of prevision and prevention activities proposed by the regional plan. Another focus concerns the immediate and technical services provided by the provincial structures. The municipalities have the same competencies as the provinces in addition to providing first aid during the emergency phase.

The complexity of the structure of civil protection should be considered according to Constitutional Law no. 3/2001 and Constitutional Article no. 118, which determined the administrative function of municipalities and other institutional administrations on the basis of the subsidiarity, differentiation, and appropriateness principles.

Finally, the last law regarding the Civil Protection Service was Law no. 100/2012. It presents some modifications to the Civil Protection Service law passed in 1992 but maintains the basic principles. The main differences are the following:

- Establishes a time limit for intervention and a state of emergency of 90 days after the impact.
- Limits events, defined previously as, "natural calamities, catastrophes or other events, which for intensity and extent, require extraordinary means/resources and powers," to a specific and detailed timeline.
- Focuses more attention on activities to guarantee risk mitigation as well as prevision and prevention activities.
- Changes the definition of *prevision* to "identification of possible risk scenario."
- Regarding prevention, specified nonstructural activities such as warning, emergency planning, and training.
- Requires that the civil protection plan be integrated with the environmental management plan of the regional agencies.
- Focuses more attention on economic resources to guarantee efficacious management after an emergency.
- Excludes competencies related to "mega events," which, during the few years before the law, caused problems with management and identification of social actors who should be involved in their control.
- Includes more structured legislation during the period of the intervention.
- Relates rescue activities more to an integrated and coordinated system of intervention.

– Requires that a state of emergency be declared in the imminence of the critical event.
– Changes the activities of the prefect and her/his coordination action with local, regional, and central organizations.

This law highlighted different sections of the National Civil Protection Service: economic, legislative, and organizational. The two most important differences in the context of this book are represented by the different perceptions of risk mitigation and the exclusion of mega events. The first focuses attention on the possibility of proactive behavior at all levels of emergency and disaster management, including the population and its need for training and information. The second is a future challenge for the role of civil protection in the emergency and disaster management process. Excluding mega events from the competencies of the Civil Protection Service means that it is necessary to consider other agencies that could be used during these particular events.

4.5 Organization of the Civil Protection Service

In Italy the Civil Protection System resembles a pyramidal structure. The historical, political, and legislative analysis concentrated on the change between the first representation of the civil protection system as a centralized affair. With the coming of the new century, however, other institutional, private, and public members participate according to the sociological process of the social inclusion of various subjects within the civil protection scenario.

The first member of the Civil Protection Service is the citizen. Citizens are the base of this figure and has the primary responsibility to educate, inform, and train themselves, especially with regard to warning and prevention activities. Because of the identification of the community and citizens as fundamental and active members of any civil protection system, it is on this institutional, legal, and cultural basis that specific training courses should be proposed to the population. An interesting example of this form of participation is the Home Office guidelines for the recovery and reconstruction phase. The ultimate aim of this activity should be not only the physical reconstruction of the community affected by a disaster but also a symbolic reconstruction of social ties. This activity becomes possible only when the following actions occur:

– Economic resources management.
– Resources management, in particular the role of voluntary services.
– Response to the needs of the community.
– Development of strategies.

In relation to the citizen is the base of the civil protection system, particular attention should be focused on voluntary services activities as linking activities between citizens and public administrations. The specific role of voluntary services and their important presence during all phases of crisis and disaster management are discussed later. The best anthropological and philosophical paradigm is the man as an open system, which views man as, for example, the citizen in an emergency linked with the community and the local administration as a first level of disaster management practice.

The second member involved in the Civil Protection System is the local administration or municipality. Italy has a long tradition of municipalities and their activities. At this level the mayor is the institutional figure with formal authority of civil protection at the local level. The mayor's specific competencies concern civil protection issues in terms of first aid organization and includes understanding whether the event can be managed with local resources or if more help from the other institutional levels of civil protection is needed and. If crisis and disaster management can be managed at a local level, the mayor has the tasks of coordinating first aid and urgent interventions and advising the prefect and provincial authorities.

Legislative Decree no. 112/98 affirms the functions of local administrations, which include the following:

- Realizing, at a local level, specific activities of civil protection, such as prevision and prevention.
- Considering all measure of the management of emergencies and calamitous events.
- Predisposition of local and interlocal emergency plans (also referring to the cooperative forms as established in legislative Decree no. 267/2000).
- Providing first aid and urgent interventions to the population.
- Controlling first aid and urgent interventions.
- Managing the participation of local or interlocal voluntary services.

Furthermore, the local administration is responsible for campaigns providing information about specific risks at local level that are of interest to the population. In this context, particular importance has been given to the evaluation of specific vulnerabilities (see Chap. 3) and their presence in the system. The importance of mapping specific vulnerabilities at the local level could create deeper knowledge in terms of prevision and prevention activities.

Overall, the civil protection plan at the local level represents the fundamental operative instrument that allows efficacious and coordinated management of emergencies and critical events.

Another member that has an important role in this organizational context is the figure of the prefect. The territorial context here is the province, and the competencies attributed to the prefect are the control of the provision of first aid during critical events and of the implementation of provincial civil protection plans. The prefect also informs the Civil Protection Department, the president of the Regional Committee, and the Regional Director of Civil Protection and Fire Control in the Ministry of the Interior. The prefect has the unitary responsibility to activate interventions at a local level and control their implementation. In extremely serious events, when a state of emergency is declared, the prefect works as the authority in the commission of the Presidency of the Council of Ministries. For temporary organization of rescue services, the prefect can use the prefecture and its members with the aim of crisis and emergency management. Finally, the figure of the prefect represents the integration, at a provincial level, of the first-level organizations for emergency management and coordinates all territorial levels and the practical interventions required in a crisis or emergency.

The province supplies provincial emergency plans and collaborates with the prefect and region according to the principles of solidarity, collaboration, and subsidiarity. In the field of civil protection the regions have important competencies, such as:

- Preparing prevision and prevention programs according to national guidelines
- Performing urgent actions in cases of crisis –events which, by their nature and their typical characteristics – require coordinated action from members and administrations, including, if necessary, the National Fire Guard
- Following guidelines for the preparation of emergency plans to enable more coordinated intervention at different levels
- Providing all interventions necessary for the recovery phase in areas stricken by a calamitous event
- Perform competencies regarding voluntary services, the associations, and their coordination

It is important to remember the constitutional principles, which should be an institutional and practical guide for all interventions and be acted upon by all different levels of public administration.

The final level to be analyzed is represented by the Civil Protection Department, which is the central member of this system. It coordinates and organizes all other members involved in civil protection issues. Law no. 401/2001 highlights the operative and technical activities of the Civil Protection Department during the first phase of an intervention. Interventions should be provided with respect to all other members involved and their specific competencies and functions and according to the criteria for the best use of necessary resources.

The process of communication represents a fundamental issue to take into consideration for crisis and disaster management at all institutional levels. In particular, the communication process in a crisis and disaster context concerns three different levels, which should be balanced for an adequate response to crisis and disaster:

- Institutional level and its legal and political framework
- Operative and technical level
- Communication link between institutions and the population at risk

Regarding this legal and organizational framework, another basilar law is Law no. 225/1992, described earlier in this chapter, which established the central members of the Italian Civil Protection Service:

- National Council of Civil Protection
- National Commission for Prevision and Prevention of big risks
- Operative Committee of Civil Protection

Other important member of the Italian Civil Protection Service are:

- National Fire Department
- Military
- Police
- Italian State Forestry Corps
- National scientific research groups
- Geophysics National Institute and other research institutions
- Italian Red Cross
- National Health Service
- Voluntary services
- Italian Alpine Troops
- National Technical Services

The Italian Civil Protection Service is involved in the administration and operative coordination between all members who participate in civil protection activities. Remember that the issue of civil protection is not a ministerial topic but is shared among different members belonging to various institutions, the private sector, and voluntary services.

The practical instruments used by the Italian Civil Protection Service to coordinate and effectively manage crises and disasters are diverse, for example, the agreement as explained by Law no.112/1998 and accords within Law no. 241/1990. More recently, this agreement has proved to be an advantage and a practical tool because it seems more effective in its aim of balancing and integrating all the different members involved in civil protection activities.

The presentation of the structure of the Italian civil protection system, starting with the important value and fundamental function attributed to the individual citizen, highlights the attention on the general issue of safety, represented as an argument shared among different members, institutions, and people and which needs to be considered from a particular point of view for better crisis and disaster management.

4.6 Activities and Instruments of Civil Protection

The activities of civil protection have as their focus the calamitous events that are possible or that have already occurred. Italian disaster management theories are used to distinguish three different critical events:

1. Simple event: natural events or events caused by human actions, which can be coped with by the resources present in a single local administration through regular procedures.
2. Complex event: events that, by their nature, extent, and intensity, need a coordinated intervention from many administrations through regular procedures.

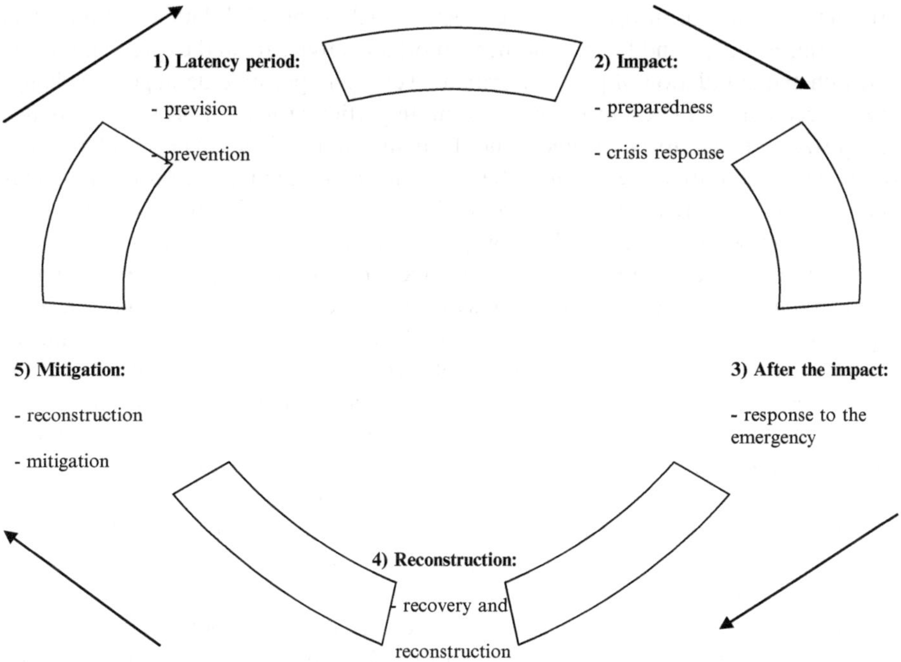

Fig. 4.1 The circle of disaster based on and adapted by Marincioni (2003)

3. Extraordinary event: natural calamities, terrorist attacks, or other events that, by their nature, extent, and intensity, need extraordinary instruments, resources, and power to cope with them.

The method of disaster management considered, such as emergency planning, is traditionally characterized by five phases; there have been many discussions about this argument and its definition over the years (Neal 1997). In this context, a general, common timeline that is also specific to the Italian civil protection system is presented.

1. Prevision and prevention
2. Warning
3. Impact
4. Rescue
5. Recovery

This process can also be seen within the circle of disaster proposed by Marincioni (2003) and adapted me (Fig. 4.1). The first phase is prevision and prevention. Prevision is characterized as a logical moment and cognitive activity; prevention represents operative output and specification. Prevision aims to identify areas that may be at risk when related to a specific risk or possible disaster. For this reason it is supported by an information service that must be updated and used to produce technical "risk maps." Data and information are developed through technological programs and useful information is collected, such as general data about a critical event, places, dates, and facts. Another important activity related to prevision is the research and simulation of possible critical events and possible damage and changing effects that could be caused by an event, in particular natural ones. It could also categorize an event, its occurrence, and its main characteristics. The simulation is a fundamental activity in developing the risk maps and planning for prevention. This is an activity directly connected with prevision. In fact, according to findings from the prevision phase, it is possible to propose some preventive strategies.

Prevention concentrates on calamitous phenomena, meaning the representation of a fact that can be understood in terms of time, space, and its own process according to qualitative and quantitative variations. These phenomena could be spontaneous or stirred up by the social dynamics of a constructed reality. A critical event is specific calamitous phenomenon, and for this reason it is included within the prevention phase. This activity involves studying and determining the causes of calamitous phenomena. Prevention is formed by all activities that impede the damage caused to or negative effects felt by the community affected by a disaster. Prevention does not have the ambitious aim of impeding damage completely; instead, it aims to limit and diminish the negative effects caused by a disaster.

The major portion of prevention in the civil protection area should be done by the regions, according to their knowledge of the environment, the population, and their specific risks. In this context the concept of risk is divided into two fundamental parts: (1) the probability of event occurring (i.e., a probabilistic approach related to an ecological approach); and (2) the extent of the damage (a technical evaluation with the aim of connecting, for example, the possible natural risk and the socio-urban characteristics of a specific area). It is important to consider that prevention activities include:

- Prevision and risk evaluation
- Elaborating an emergency plan
- Providing training and update meetings for expert personnel
- Training the vulnerable population and disseminating preventive and civil protection culture

For this reason, the primary action of civil protection is the role of municipalities.

The next phase is the warning. A warning is developed over a short time, according to the situation, and it could coincide with the third phase – impact. An alert is a specific instrument that enables the evacuation of the area and the displacement of people at risk and applies all possible safety strategies during an impact. During this phase all emergency plans are applied after the event is evaluated in terms of its nature, intensity, and extent.

The impact is the central moment of the critical event and lasts some seconds. During this phase the system is in crisis and latent vulnerabilities appear. During impact, particular attention should be focused on the behavior of the people involved. Sociological and psychological studies have observed two different types of behavior during impact: (1) feelings such as sorrow, anger, bafflement, helplessness; and (2) feelings such as solidarity and generosity and prosocial attitudes.

Based on a sociological perspective, the organization of rescue activities and the helping relationships that take place in these peculiar moments can be analyzed through two different levels. The first level includes the first aid offered by the people involved and other victims as first responders. The second level is represented by the aid offered by institutional agencies and administrations that have efficacious and effective characteristics, technical, and technological means adequate enough to be applied in a crisis scenario. In the majority of critical events in Italy, the first institutional and organizational aid is provided by the Italian Red Cross, the Fire Department (urgent technical rescue), the police force, and civil protection volunteers. It is important to understand that this is not a fixed procedure; it is flexible according to the contextual variables of the critical event. The rescue services are useful and efficacious depending on an information system that enables coordination and good communication processes. This last is fundamental in both the prevention and crisis and management phases.

The last phase includes overcoming the emergency and reconstruction. The final aim is to reestablish the social, environmental, economic, and political balance destroyed during the impact of the critical event; this is basilar for the reconstruction of the community affected by the disaster.

During the past 20/20 years, the attention of authorities has been oriented toward the competencies and functions of coordination, which is indispensable for overcoming the critical event and for evaluating the possible damage, the solutions, and the necessary aid. In this moment, the activity of coordination is restored at a central level and is not delegated to only specific functions and tasks.

The principal instrument of all these activities is the civil protection plan, which exists at local, provincial, and regional levels. The civil protection plan must always be created, although many times no critical event occurs. This plan is based on the possible characteristics of a critical event related to the territorial, social, economic, and political indicators of to the specific area considered. It presents strategies to cope with a crisis and disaster and the response to them, as well as the operative techniques, procedures, and interventions to be applied in case of emergency. The general aim of these activities is the safeguarding of human life and, if possible, cultural and architectural heritage.

The plan is made up of three elements: (1) the scenario; (2) strategies; and (3) an intervention model. The first element describes the characteristics of the event and its probable process and damage. It is a dynamic activity, even if it is an internal structure.

There are three types of phenomena:

- Known and quantifiable phenomena (most in this category are natural events)
- Known and not quantifiable phenomena
- Unknown phenomena that can be considered rare events because of their dimension and their intensity

Furthermore, the civil protection plan should be drawn up in line with some general principles:

- Preserve the principles of coordination, solidarity, and subsidiarity.
- Keep procedures simple.
- Identify specific competencies and functions.
- Allow for operative flexibility to take into account any new element, which is inevitable in an emergency or crisis scenario.

The emergency plan should be written according to the prevision and preventive indications at a central level and should contain all information regarding the territorial area involved (physical processes, past phenomena, possibility of next phenomena, resources). Maps should always be included both in the elaboration phase and during the utilization of the plans to limit the territorial area at risk and to facilitate the coordination of rescue teams.

On a practical level, the plan is divided into three parts:

1. General/informative: all the useful information about the territorial area potentially at risk is collected in this part.
2. Planning and the identification of objectives that are fundamental for this response and to have an organized system.
3. Model of intervention complete with tasks, functions, and competencies.

Finally, it is important remember that the plan must always be updated and evaluated on the basis of territorial indicators, population, and other general characteristics of the area potentially at risk.

4.7 Civil Defense: A Diverse Approach for an Organized Response to an Emergency

In Italy, civil defense is considered a diverse approach to an organized response to an emergency because of its major connection with the military; even if civil defense and civil protection are different with regard to organizations, competencies, functions, activities, strategies, and operative methods, they are simultaneously present in cases of crisis and emergency (Alexander 2002). Civil defense is represented within the general national defense. National defence has a military force (military defense) and a civil force (civil defense). The activities of national defense are related to the structures of the State, and they guarantee the integrity and safety of the nation at every level (political, military, and economic). This is possible through its three fundamental components: (1) military defense; (2) civil defense; and (3) civil-military cooperation.

Civil defense is defined as actions with the aim of national security in all emergency situations caused by an aggressive attack on the nation. The historical process of civil defense can be divided into three parts: World Wars I and II, the Cold War, and the origin of nuclear power (as a weapon of mass destruction and not as possibility for development). In both world wars, civil defense was understood as defense against air attacks, whereas during the Cold War and the nuclear period it has been recognized as a fundamental activity for maintaining and recovering the organizational structure of a nation stricken by an attack, through directional functions, coordination, and communication systems.

In Italy there is no specific legislation on the issue of civil defense; all laws seem fragmentary. Legislative Decree no. 300/1999, modified with Law no. 401/2001, established the competencies and authorities for these functions. The competency and responsibility in terms of civil defense is attributed to the Minister of Interior, who has the task of guaranteeing security and public order using all available resources to achieve these objectives.

At a technical and operative level, the Fire Department responsible for this issue and must be present in any crisis or emergency caused by terrorist or military attacks with or without the use of nonconventional weapons. Directive no. 6/2002, "Organization of the response by the Fire Department to chemical, biological, nuclear and radiological emergencies," considers more adequate organization and procedures in case of these peculiar emergencies. In particular, the Fire Department takes part in a context where nonconventional weapons have been used through the intervention of a group called the CRNB (chemical, radioactive, nuclear, bacteriological group). It is a group that specializes in these forms of attacks and it provides urgent technical rescue through the decontamination and circumscription of the possible contaminated area. The CRNB is organized into four components:

- Basilar team
- Provincial team
- Regional team (firemen and experts)
- Mobile support tool as a model of mobilization

The organizational model of these specialists is based upon three elements: training, procedures, and equipment.

According to this brief overview, civil defense is directly connected with national defense, and it uses the same instruments and operative tools specific to military strategies. The fundamental aims of civil defense are:

- Maintaining all activities to guarantee institutional and administrative continuity at both a central and local level
- Safeguarding financial, economic, logistic, and productive organizations
- Guaranteeing the protection of and mediating resistance among the population
- Supporting the military defense

The activities of civil defense can be distinguished at two levels.

1. Internal: the aim of civil defense is the protection and safety of the population from external attacks, institutional continuity, and the guarantee of the security and continuity of business within the nation.

2. International: guarantees the national contribution to collective action during the management of an international crisis. The final aim here is the creation of an effective state of "peace" that can develop opportunities for countries in a permanent state of war. Specifically, civil defense has an active role in international collaboration within North Atlantic Treaty Organization and the European community.

It is interesting that this book considers the context and competencies of civil defense according to contemporary societies, which are characterized by urgency, uncertainty, and geopolitical instability, and can often determine internal and/or external crises involving telecommunication systems, critical infrastructures, and international networks, with the consequences of both global crises and local emergencies.

International terrorism has focused attention on vulnerability and its presence at multiple levels – political, economic, organizational and social – within a nation.

Accordingly, civil defense should be understood within the more complex organization of national defense. Proposing the decentralization of some concrete institutional issues seems to be inappropriate in the case of civil defense and its competencies, functions, and model of organization.

4.8 Two Systems of Organizational Response to an Emergency: Analysis and Evaluation

This analysis of the civil protection system and the civil defense system has been possible by taking into account some useful indicators:

- Organization and structure
- Competencies and functions
- Lead authority
- Roles and activities
- Instruments for intervention
- Centralization versus decentralization
- Subsidiarity (vertical/horizontal) versus authoritarian internal coordination
- Voluntary services versus professional careers
- Different presence of these actors on the territory
- Different historical moments for the development of the analysis and evaluation of crisis and disaster response
- Different possibilities for active participation by citizens
- Strategies for prevention

The first indicator concerns the organization and the structure of analysis and evaluation response models. The civil protection system is organized along the lines of a decentralized logic and structure. In fact, it has been classified as a participative issue between the State and other administrations situated at different levels.

According to this vision, it is possible to consider the constitutional principles of adequacy, collaboration, and solidarity. It is also interesting to remember that civil protection is an issue within civil rights and that it is focused on sustainable development and the concrete possibility of progress for the population and the nation in general. In this case, the decentralization logic is not only used for the institutional activities and planning at a central and local level but also is considered within the logic of major knowledge about the territory, its characteristics, and the population that lives there.

Civil protection activities are articulated according to the Augustus method, which schedules the phases of prevision and prevention with the aim of guaranteeing adequate knowledge and awareness about the characteristics of the territory potentially at risk. The territory represents the contextual and physical context within which the civil protection system works to achieve its own objectives.

Instead, the civil defense system is a centralized structure, and the level of administrative and institutional agencies is limited to the provincial level and the figure of the prefect. Civil defense is exclusively an issue of the central State. The context of activity of the civil defense system can be represented by the political, economic, social, and infrastructural relationships that are of interest to the security of a nation and its institutional and administrative continuity. Civil defense as civil protection is interested in the territorial issue, but not at an environmental and spatial level; instead it refers to its geopolitical meaning.

For this reason, all prevision and prevention activities are located within simulation models and training experiences. The gap here is in terms of predictability according to scientific elaboration during, for example, for a natural disaster. Civil defense is deeply involved within national and international relationships and the specific political, economic, and social relations the nation has with foreign countries. Regarding the importance of relationships within the issue of a terrorist attack and the possibility of prevention, according to this specific argument, civil defense does not allow the active participation of citizens in the case of such emergencies because of its specific logic and organizational model.

The second indicator regards competencies and functions typical of these analysis and evaluation crisis and disaster management systems. The civil protection service, as mentioned earlier, identifies its own competencies and functions in Law no. 225/1992. The functions and competencies of the civil protection service should be understood within the context of other constitutional laws, specifically with regard for the principles of subsidiarity, solidarity, and collaboration.

At a legislative level, the civil defence system seems less structured than civil protection. In fact, the normative reference to civil defense is Legislative Decree no. 300/99, modified with Law no. 401/2001. It is necessary to think carefully about the fact that these laws are recent, and this affects civil defense in two ways. First, as mentioned, civil defense is a part of national defense within a military structure. Civil defense has changed in the past 10 years, and it is developing because of the major availability of other forms of structure and participation. Second, the year of the law – 2001 – is very revealing. The terrorist attacks on the U.S.A. have

Table 4.1 Civil protection and civil defence systems and their lead authorities

System	Lead authorities
Civil protection	Presidency of the Council of Ministries
National defense	Department of Defense
Civil defense	Department of the Interior

completely changed the way of thinking about political and economic relationships among nations as well as national operative and technical issues.

The third aspect to be considered concerns the lead authority in a political and administrative context. The lead authority of the civil protection service is the Department of Civil Protection within the Presidency of the Council of Ministries, and so it is not considered a ministerial issue. The lead authority of civil defense, on the other hand, is the Minister of the Interior, who during emergency situations must maintain and guarantee public order and national security and uses resources to achieve these objectives. These authorities must coordinate of all useful activities and actions in a unique way to achieve the objectives of the different organizations. For a better understanding of this particular organization see Table 4.1.

Analyzing the roles and the activities of these two organized systems (the civil protection service and civil defense) is possible by the following considerations. Civil protection has a role during prevision, prevention, rescue, and recovery. It is interested in risk for the first two phases and then in crisis and emergency actions. Its must look at different timing of the phases and various technical and operative strategies. Civil defense has an active role; in particular, the Fire Department is part of national defense and has been assigned to emergency and crisis situations or disasters caused by human action, for example, terrorist attacks.

It is possible to make analyze these systems at two different levels. At the macro level, both systems are interested in risks, emergency, and crisis, whereas at the micro level they are different with regard to lead agencies, national authorities, and the types of interventions they provide during critical events and according to their particular competencies and functions. The decision to decentralize the Civil Protection Service was possible by taking into consideration the necessity of its presence in local areas and the issues that it must face. In particular, the Service is involved in natural risk management and, because of its characteristics, its presence has been logically organized at national, regional, provincial, and local levels.

Furthermore, considering prevision and prevention activities in Italy, we can find examples of scientific centers built near an area at major risk, such as the earthquake center in Gorizia or the volcanic center near Etna and Vesuvio. This is a strategic choice, allowing the study of natural phenomena and the monitoring of their evolution. Remember that, as members of the National Civil Protection Service, these are scientific institutes that can offer information and data to the Civil Protection Department with the aim of monitoring and alerting of activity. This is a necessary interconnection that guarantees the general aim of the National Civil Protection Service, that is, to safeguard life and maintain the integrity of the environment and cultural heritage.

Civil defense is based on a centralized organization because it is part of national defense and the Minister of the Interior has competencies for civil defense.

It also important to note that civil defense, as represented by the Fire Department, is divided at regional and provincial levels.

In the past few years there have been proposals for the creation of the Fire Service at a local level within municipalities. This is how things are organized in, for example, France, and there depends on the size of cities and municipalities. This system is interesting for the Italian Civil Protection Service and its necessary risk communication and early warning activities.

An important piece of data, in addition to territorial levels, is the number of people that inhabit a place. This is a core concept if connected with the importance of information and communication regarding best and safe behavior in cases of emergency and crisis. Risk communication should refer to all possible phases of a disaster, starting with the preventive phase. This practice must also be considered regarding the simplification of rescue and recovery intervention; the population involved in the critical event should be able to activate the self-protection strategies and the specialist teams should focus on operative and practical interventions.

In this context, the decrease of distance among the population – the citizens and the operative personnel – is important to consider. The specific and professional competencies of firemen and civil protection people must be maintained, but it is also important to create some sort of resilience behavior among the people who need to be able to face and cope with the primary phase of an emergency or disaster. This is possible only with the implementation of communication activities between the local and regional authorities and the population potentially at risk.

In line with this, it is important to consider the importance of schools and their role in adequate risk communication for children and adolescents, taking into account their particular age and personal characteristics. In Italy, this information process was created following the industrial accidents near Seveso in Northern Italy in 1986 and directives that have been developed for this kind of accident at a European level.

Several activities must be repeated, depending on the risk being communicated and the information available to the population at risk. Many inadequacies are evident, and the approach to this core issue is different between the north and the south of Italy, even though the inadequacies are often quite similar in all regions of Italy. No systematic processes regarding risk communication have been created. This could be considered proof of the willingness to maintain the people's vulnerability and not consider the possibilities of resilience among the population.

Another significant element of the two systems – analyze and evaluate – is the subsidiarity principle and its application at both vertical and horizontal levels. Civil protection in Italy is a decentralized issue, and so subsidiarity is present at a vertical level depending on its organization (state, region, province, and municipality) and at a horizontal level in terms of the Civil Protection Voluntary Service. Also, because of its military and hierarchical components and because in the civil defense system there is no voluntary service (it is advantaged by being composed of professional people), civil defense represents the vertical subsidiarity.

This last aspect, the presence or absence voluntary service, is an important question within the analysis of this dual organized system to crisis and emergency response.

The Italian Civil Protection Service has volunteers as a fundamental member of its interventions. This is particularly important because part of this research is based on an online questionnaire sent to civil protection volunteers to define their characteristics in order to understand a possible professional disaster resilience.

Italian civil protection volunteers are organized in groups at the municipal, provincial, and regional levels, but we cannot forget the role of the "independent" association outside of the institutional network. Specifically, voluntary organizations that have civil protection activities in their statute are recognized as members of the National Civil Protection Service at national, regional, provincial, and local levels. Civil protection volunteers can be identified as people who perform particular activities, such as:

- Organizing all useful knowledge about specific risks in terms of social networks and within the preventive phase
- Making the population aware about potential risks in the area
- Supporting study and research activities in the civil protection field
- Creating activities for future civil protection volunteers
- Disseminating knowledge of civil protection activities among the population

It is important to highlight the difference between civil protection volunteers and professional civil defense personnel. Strictly speaking, the former are not professional personnel with the obvious characteristics of this profession; however; they carry out professional activities during times of peace and during emergencies.

The Civil Protection Voluntary Service focuses on the organization of and the response by civil society in cases of emergency. This situation is created by the need of some citizens who, without specific reasons and motives, decide to organize groups and associations that are formally recognized and are established by law and institutional agencies. The ambivalence of the Civil Protection Voluntary Service is clear. On one hand, it can be considered a limitation of operative, urgent, and technical interventions because they require more advanced professional skills. On the other hand, it is an indispensable resource that can contribute in the rescue and recovery phases, where the focus should not be on the technical aspects but on relational and interpersonal competencies.

The analysis of this dual system of organized response to crisis also concerns the historical period of their founding. In particular, civil defense was founded because of critical events caused by human actions: World Wars I and II, the Cold War, and, more recently, international terrorism. Instead, civil protection was started during the development of civil societies and new reflections on a fundamental aspect, such as safety in welfare states.

To conclude this analysis, the last elements to be considered are the different possibilities of participation by the population, which can be either involved or uninvolved in a crisis or emergency. Because of its structural characteristics, the Civil Protection Service seems more open to the diverse participation of the civilian population during the phases of a crisis, whereas civil defense excludes any participation of the civilian population because of its own organizations, aim, structure, and personnel. This crucial difference is understandable in light of the operative and strategic levels of the civil defense response and because the civilian population is considered to be a vulnerable element that needs to be safeguarded, although this is not the first aim of civil defense.

Another issue is that, in the civil protection field, prevention and technical operative actions must be done during the preventive phase. Instead, in the civil defense field, prevention does not exist in this way but through simulations and training of professional personnel. Because of its specific characteristics, the possibility of prevention in civil defense field can be found in all international activities, such as negotiations and within geopolitical relationships. In this context, the instruments of negotiation seem to be more adaptive than other preventive strategies.

Finally, although the organization of civil defense and its aim, structures, functions, and roles are understandable, it is important to underline the necessity of more informed people even if crisis and disaster management during the primary phase is attributed to technical and operative aid. The lack of some basilar instruments in cases of crisis and emergency would, for example, leave people and infrastructure open to vulnerability: the civilian population should be involved in some aspects in this social process, where many social and personal identities with peculiar needs, sense-making, and meaning-making meet.

4.9 Final Considerations

The analysis and comparison of the field of crisis, emergency, and disaster management has made it possible to claim that, in the case of critical events in Italy, two distinct response systems exist, and they have differences at many levels of analysis. However, it is possible to talk about a unique system of crisis and emergency response when considering the significant differences that characterize the two systems.

The field of intervention includes different organizations, institutional agencies, structures, tasks, aims, competencies, roles, and methods. This is an important point that can be useful and interesting for all the people involved in the process and its management. In particular, sometimes there is conflict and confusion around the question of who performs a specific task. Rivalry is not an occasional occurrence; instead it reflects economic, political, and institutional interests that are always present in times of crisis and emergency.

Another point of confusion is the opposite points of view of professional experts and volunteers. Integration at different levels and respect for the peculiarity of each response system – not meaning confusion or loss of specific competencies of these two systems but instead as complementary actions to do with safeguarding the population and institutional and administrative continuity – seem to be betters final goals of each system.

It seems clear that civil defense has the competence for urgent technical intervention or "the aim of national security in all emergency situations determined by acts against the Nation." Future development should be oriented to a new pervasive prevention phase including the civilian population, too. The Civil Protection Service, on the other hand, seems more closed off from European orientations and more connected with reflection about the economic, social, and political development of Italy.

Finally, the dual response system can be understood by referring to real possibilities of coordination and collaboration in cases of critical events. Coordinating activities should be of interest at all levels – political, administrative, institutional, technical, and operative – according to the guidelines represented by the collaboration and solidarity principles among all public institutions and agencies.

This theoretical and legislative analysis is fundamental for the next topic of this research, that is, the Civil Protection Voluntary Service, the possibility of professional resilience, and its future development. It is also useful at a practical level to better understand the framework within which civil protection voluntary activities and interventions take place.

Part II
Empirical Research

Chapter 5
Into the Field: Three Italian Earthquakes

Three fieldworks present the choice of earthquakes and the preexisting environmental and organizational conditions of the Umbria, Molise, and Abruzzo regions before the earthquakes. This chapter especially considers the impact phase of the earthquakes and their physical features. It also includes reflections of the personal coming of myself, as a researcher, and some considerations about these three fieldworks and the environmental and social conditions of the regions. It can be explained as a brief ethnographic approach to the fieldwork that is important for the future reflections on the sense of community, sense of place, and place attachment. Furthermore, this chapter explains fundamental ideas about social researchers and their ethics in the context of applied research within the sociology of disasters because this fieldwork made me aware of the possible distance between social researchers and earthquake victims, the social relationships among these two social actors, and the ethical questions of applied research.

5.1 Introduction

For this research, the kind of disaster to be studied was determined by following a rational and logic implications analysis. Because of personal interests and attitudes considering natural disasters as an "old" and fascinating social process, the following were not considered: technological disasters, terrorist disasters, or disasters caused by human actions.

Because of different theoretical elaboration on disaster resilience from a sociological perspective, I thought it would be better to choose at least two natural disasters. After a brief period of reflection, I chose to focus on three natural disasters to avoid the necessity of comparison in the case of two.

The kind of natural disaster to study remained the problem, and much help in this context was received from the National Civil Protection Department and its professional employees, who suggested to me the following three earthquakes in Italy:

B. Lucini, *Disaster Resilience from a Sociological Perspective*, Humanitarian Solutions in the 21st Century, DOI 10.1007/978-3-319-04738-6_5,

Umbria and Marche in 1997, Molise in 2002, and Abruzzo in 2009. I immediately liked the idea of studying these three earthquakes in Italy because of the interesting observations that I can argue from the historical point of view about the evolution of the Italian Civil Protection Service.

Once this was decided, some people told me that three earthquakes might require too much work to explore and comprehend; however, I believe that three earthquakes are the right number to proceed with in an initial exploration of a new theoretical issue and methodological framework in the sociological field.

Another remark made to me pointed out that the three regions stricken by the earthquakes are very close to each other in the same geographical area: the central region for the earthquake in Umbria and Marche and the southern regions for the Abruzzo and Molise earthquakes. In response to this point I note the substantial literature and specific research showing the particularities of each disaster, even if the regions stricken by them are close to each other.

Herein, I describe in depth the three Italian earthquakes, although I do not follow a quick, simple, or straightforward path.

5.2 The Umbria and Marche Earthquake in 1997

Umbria is one of the central regions of Italy, and it has been considered as the "green" region of Italy because of its characteristics such as a natural park, mountains, hills, and countryside. It has an old and religious, traditional way of thinking, similar to that in cities such as Assisi, Gubbio, and Perugia, to name the more important and most visited ones. In fact, Umbria is a region that is a point of reference for local handicrafts, culture, and the environment. The population as of January 1, 1997, was 816,100,[1] and its territory covers about 8,456 km^2.

Not only Umbria was stricken by the earthquake; the Marche region also incurred injuries and damage. Marche is another central region of Italy, and its landscape and cultural traditions are quite similar to those of the Umbria region. Its territory covers about 9,365.86 km^2 and the population as of January 1, 1997, was 1,442,523.

Although during the whole of 1997[2] there were earth tremors, the largest and most destructive earthquake was felt on September 26 at 2.33 a.m. It measured 5.5 (Maw) and VIII–IX on the Mercalli scale. Following the first, a second one occurred at 11.40 a.m. and was more powerful: 5.8 on the Richter scale.[3]

Regarding the first and tremendous earthquake, 11 people died and 100 were injured.

There were another two earth tremors on October 14 and April 3, 1998, but these were less intense; however, many people were frightened,

[1] This and all the other statistics come from the official site: http://demo.istat.it/ric/index.html.

[2] For a full comprehension of the facts please see this website: http://www.osservatorioricostruzione.regione.umbria.it/canale.asp?id=230.

[3] For details please look at http://www.protezionecivile.gov.it/jcms/it/terremoto_um.wp.

The municipalities at the local level in Umbria that were hit by the earthquake included Assisi, Bastia Umbra, Bevagna, Campello S. Clitunno, Cannara, Cerreto Di Spoleto, Costacciaro, Foligno, Fossato Di Vico, Gualdo Tadino, Gubbio (Fraz. Di Padule, Branca, Spada, S. Marco, Torre Calzolari, Colpalombo, Carbonesca), Montefalco, Nocera Umbra, Perugia (Fraz. Di Pianello, Castel D'arno, Ripa), Preci, Scheggia e Pascelupo, Sellano, Sigillo, Spello, Spoleto (Fraz. Di Poreta, S. Giacomo, Bazzano, Fabbreria, Silvignano, Eggi, Beroide, S.M. In Campis, S. Paolo, Protte, Campo Salese, Azzano, Camporoppolo), Trevi, Valfabbrica, Vallo Di Nera, and Valtopina. The municipalities at local level in Marche that were hit by the earthquake included Camerino, San Severino Marche, Caldarola, Visso, Fabriano, Matelica, and Pioraco e Fiuminata.

As a consequence of the earthquakes, more than 20,000 people were evacuated. After providing first aid, the next work was the construction of new, permanent housing for these people. Permanent houses were constructed in 23 municipalities in Marche and 26 municipalities in Umbria: the new urban surface was 223,000 m^2 in Marche and 933,000 m^2 in Umbria. After the emergency period and the relocation of people to their new homes, the process of reconstruction started. The process is divided into three levels: light, hard, and integrated.

What should be pointed out is the lack of a "real" civil protection system until this event. In fact, before 1997, Italian civil protection was not organized – even in the contemporary National Civil Protection Service. In that same year it was constituted by the spontaneous and heavy work of free citizens, spontaneous helpers, first responders, and volunteers and was not present at a local level as it is now. It was a voluntary service made up of civil volunteers and it was not directly connected with a structured civil protection organization.

An important aspect of this earthquake was that it also struck the important religious and artistic city of Assisi. When it occurred, the first thought was for the symbolic representation of the city, both of the population involved in the disaster and the cultural and artistic heritage, and its importance to the people living there (Miller and Rivera 2008).

After considering the general characteristics of this earthquake, I chose the specific place to go and interview people. To define the criteria of selection and the elements used to identify the location for research fieldwork, I chose to focus attention on and conduct interviews in the context and municipality most affected by the earthquake. Another factor was the availability of a facilitator to act as a middleman and contact people who would be available for interviews

In light of this, the first fieldwork was performed in Foligno and its three spatial divisions: the mountains and the zone of the epicenter, the hills, and the city. From my point of view, these spatial distinctions could give me various points of view of the same disaster but with different preliminary conditions, effects, and strategies of response.

5.2.1 My Arrival in Foligno and Its Surroundings

My sociological observations during my stay in the Umbria region were presented earlier in this chapter. Some preliminary remarks are necessary to understand better my lack of personal experience – and my surprise and astonishment at some things I did not completely understand – regarding Italy and its regions. Because of my family background I knew little about Italian cities and their surrounding areas.

Here I present the social context and the situation of getting to the field to conduct interviews with the population (see Chap. 8) as well as the methods used. Regarding the interviews, a person who works in civil protection in the Foligno municipality introduced me to three people – each of them middlemen and each in a different area mentioned earlier: mountains, hills, and city. After this first contact I was able to interview seven people:

- Two in the mountain area: Verchiano municipality
- Two in the hill area: Capodacqua municipality
- Three in the city of Foligno

The last consideration before proceeding with my first observations is that I did not expressly use the observations as methodological instruments of social science. As a sociologist, I think there is something innate and natural when we are going to a place with the specific aim of a research project. Moreover, as all researchers do, I needed to shape myself into a sort of "new" identity, as both researcher and student. I must confess that this made me anxious and nervous because I noted that a researcher and a student have a completely different influence on ordinary people. This perhaps was also the result of my own uncertainty regarding my position, and I was conscious about the chaos that it could create. In general terms, I had to try to balance these two different identities in a contemporary way, because among institutional people, a researcher is considered with more simplicity, whereas with ordinary people I had to continue with my favorite position as a PhD student. However, I think that the mixed identity of a PhD student–researcher is the most appropriate, and I believe that as sociologists we should always take into account the specific group of people we are studying.

I arrived in Verchiano, a municipality near Colfiorito is the epicenter of the earthquake. Going through these little streets, one can see the symbols of the reconstruction activities that were already present and images of what was done after the earthquake. I noticed the permanent wooden houses that had been constructed after the first impact. They shocked me because of their order and the absence of people; the inhabitants explained to me that now these houses are used only for holidays and just a few families bought them after the reconstruction phase.

I also was stunned by the spatial use of the mountains and their total independence from the city of Foligno; in fact, all primary services are available, and I felt a sense of a closed and defined community. Maybe it was for this reason that what remained to be reconstructed after 14 years was only a few buildings because of the poor choice of construction firms. Even if I was always conscious of the dramatic experiences of the local population, I also felt the return to normality or, maybe more precisely, a more organized style of life.

The other place where I went was Capodacqua, a municipally in the hills. Here all the houses have been reconstructed, and only some needed new more work on them because of the choice of construction firms, as in Verchiano.

Capodacqua is almost the same as Verchiano, suggesting to me the closeness of the community and networks with other people. All services are available, and you can see the signs of complete reconstruction, even if there is a universal presence of a new style of life, social change, and the absence of children – there are fewer than in previous years because families are moving nearer to the city of Foligno.

First impressions, however, made me aware of good strategies of response and reconstruction after the earthquake. Also, according to the next analysis, I think that the time of this earthquake should be considered fundamental because it occurred 14 years ago.

The last place I visited was Foligno city, and the people I met lived in the city's downtown area. It is characterized by a network of little streets and houses that are not accessible by car. This is the basilar characteristic to understanding the population and its changes in the past 15 years . My personal observations focused on this physical and structural particularity that has influenced the reconstruction phase and the first aid provided.

Another thing to point out is the spatial dispersion and the difficulty connecting the downtown of the city with its surroundings. It seemed me less closed as a community, perhaps because of the large presence of strangers in the city and their presence when the earthquake occurred. This spatial structure of the downtown area made me doubtful regarding the possibility of another earthquake and whether it would be possible to help the people living in those streets, although the inhabitants told me that all the houses were built 600 years ago with large, strong walls.

Finally, as I mentioned before, Foligno city seems to me a city with the same problems as all others in this period: increasing urbanization, change of inhabitants, and movement from the downtown to the countryside and vice versa.

The possibility of localizing my first fieldwork into three different levels of space allowed me to analyze the same earthquake and its impact at the community level, on spatial considerations, and on different institutional and cultural organizations within these three areas that were affected by the Umbria earthquake in 1997.

5.3 The Molise Earthquake in 2002

Molise is one of the smallest regions of Italy, after Valle d'Aosta. Its population comprises about 319,611 inhabitants and its territory is about 4.438 km^2 in size. The earthquake occurred on October 31, 2002, at 11.33 a.m., and it measured 5.4 on the

Richter scale and VIII–IX on the Mercalli scale. The inhabitants present in 2002, at the moment of the earthquake, numbered 320,467.[4]

The epicenter was located between the municipalities of Bonefro and Montorio in Frentani and Santa Croce di Magliano in the province of Campobasso. The municipalities at the local level in the province of Campobasso and Molise that were hit by the earthquake included Bonefro, Campolieto, Campomarino, Casacalenda, Castelbottaccio, Castellino del Biferno, Castelmauro, Colletorto, Guardialfiera, Guglionesi, Larino, Limosano, Lucito, Lupara, Macchia Valfortore, Matrice, Montagano, Montelongo, Montenero di Bisaccia, Montorio nei Frentani, Morrone del Sannio, Petacciato, Portocannone, Provvidenti, Ripabottoni, Rotello, San Giacomo degli Schiavoni, San Giovanni in Galdo, San Giuliano di Puglia, San Martino in Pensilis, Sant'Elia a Pianisi, Santa Croce di Magliano, Termoli, and Ururi. The municipalities hit in the provinces of Foggia and Puglia were Carlantino, Casalnuovo Monterotaro, Celenza Valfortore, Foggia, Lesina, Lucera, San Paolo di Civitate, San Severo, Serracapriola, Torremaggiore, Sannicandro Garganico, Carpino, and a small part of Volturara Appula.

Specifically, we can consider the following list of intensities of the earthquake on the Mercalli scale associated with the municipalities involved:

- Grade VIII–IX: San Giuliano di Puglia
- Grade VII: Bonefro, Casalnuovo Monterotaro, Castellino del Biferno, Ripabottoni, Santa Croce di Magliano
- Grade VI–VII: Colletorto, Montelongo
- Grade VI: Casacalenda, Larino, Montorio nei Frentani, Morrone del Sannio, Pietramontecorvino, Provvidenti, Rotello, Ururi
- Grade V–VI: Campodipietra, Campolieto, Carlantino, Casalvecchio di Puglia, Castellino Nuovo, Castelnuovo della Daunia, Celenza Valfortore, Chieuti, Guardialfiera, Limosano, Lucito, Lupara, Macchia Valfortore, Monacilioni, Montagano, Petrella Tifernina, Poggio Imperiale, San Martino in Pensilis, San Paolo Civitade, Sant'Elia a Pianisi, Toro, Tufara
- Grade V: Acquaviva Collecroce, Apricena, Campobasso, Castelbottaccio, Castelmauro, Civitacampomarano, Gambatesa, Guglionesi, Lesina, Lucera, Matrice, Montecilfone, Motta Montecorvino, Palata, Pietracatella, Ripalimosani, San Giovanni in Galdo, San Marco La Catola, San Severo, Sant'Angelo Limosano, Serracapriola, Termoli, Torremaggiore, Volturara Appula

Thirty people died, in particular, 27 children in their school together with their teacher; 100 people were injured and 2,925 people were displaced. The death of 27 children caused the most damage to this community, not in terms of physical damage, but instead according to a symbolic and emotional loss: they were children enjoying a normal day of school. This is an incredible thing to comprehend.

[4] Data from www.demo.istat.it.

5.3.1 *My Arrival in San Giuliano di Puglia, Casacalenda, Larino*

Curious as usual, I decided to go to Molise to interview earthquake victims, and I started my observation the first day I arrived. It is important to specify that I arrived in Casacalenda because it can be reached by public transport; all other places can be reached only by car, and one or two can be reached by a daily bus. As a sociologist, the mobility issue posed interesting questions about life there and the use of territory and space. In fact, my first impression was one of incredible isolation – the nearest city to Casacalenda is Termoli, which is 1 h away by train.

So, when I arrived, I started my observations, and something important happened to me. I felt myself deeply observed by the people when I walked down the street. I found that it was not possible to disappear or seem to be one of them. It was clear that I was a stranger, and they did nothing to overcome this situation or make me feel me more comfortable. I think this was one of the reasons that the interviews became so difficult: the people were distrustful and suspicious.

My impression of Casacalenda, Larino, and San Giuliano di Puglia and a general note about the Molise region is the large movement of people from these small places. Families leaving has the direct consequence of increasing the number of older people with all their specific needs. All these places gave me the impression of wanting to be separate from the rest of the world, in a sort of defense of their own place and territory.

5.4 The Abruzzo Earthquake in 2009

Abruzzo is a region in Southern Italy. Its population in 2009, the year of the earthquake, was about 1,334,675, and its territory measures 10,753 km^2. The first strong shock occurred on April, 6, 2009 at 3.32 a.m., with a 5.9 magnitude on the Richter scale and 6.3 (Maw) and VIII/IX on the Mercalli scale. The epicenter was between the villages of Roio Colle and Genzano e Collefracido and some villages in central Italy. During the earthquake, 308 people died and 1,600 people were injured. During the following 48 h, there were 256 aftershocks: 150 occurred on April 7 alone.

According to the Italian Civil Protection Department, 48,818 people were displaced on August 9: 19,973 went to 137 tent cities (5,029 tents), 19,149 went to hotels, and 9,696 went to private houses. In addition, we must not forget the 273 people who displaced themselves into 9 spontaneous camps.

The municipalities and cities stricken by this earthquake can be distinguished according to the province:

- L'Aquila: Acciano, Beffi, San Lorenzo, Roccapreturo, Succiano, Barete, Barisciano and surroundings, Picenze, Bugnara, Calascio, Cansano, Capestrano, Capitignano, Cararpelle Calvisio, Castel del Monte, Castel di Ieri, Castelvecchio

Calvisio, Castelvecchio Sebequo, Celano, Cerchio, Collarmele, Corfinio, Fagnano, Fontecchio, Fossa, Goriano Sicoli, L'Aquila and its surroundings, Arischia, Bazzano, Camarda, Bagno, Civita, Menzano, Moticchio, Onna, Pescara, Paganica, Poggio di Roio, Preturo, San Gregorio, San Gregorio Magno, Tempera, Lucoli, Collimento, Francolisco, Magliano de' Marsi, Molina Aterno, Montereale, Ocre, Ofena, Pizzoli, Poggio Picenze, Prata d'Ansidonia, Pratola Peligna, Raiano, Rocco di Cambio, Rocca di Mezzo, San Demetrio ne' Vestini, San Pio delle Camere, Sant'Eusanio Forconese, Santo Stefano di Sessanio, Scoppito, Scurcola Marsicana, Secinaro, Sulmona, Tione, Tornimparte, Villa Sant'Angelo
- Teramo: Bisenti, Campli, Colledara, Montorio al Vomano, Nereto, Tours, Penna Sant'Andrea, Teramo
- Chieti: Chieti, Fara Filiorum Petri, Francavilla al Mare, Guardiagrele, Miglianico, Ripa Teatina
- Pescara: Brittoli, Bussi sul Tirino, Castiglione a Casauria, Civitella Casanova and surroundings, Farindola, Loreto Aprutino, Pescara, Pianella, Penne, Popoli, Torre de' Passeri
- Roma: Montelanico, Roma
- Rieti: Antrodoco, Rieti, Borgorose, Fiamignano, Pescorocchiano
- Frosinone: Fiuggi, Giuliano di Roma, Sora Frosinone, Isola del Liri, Veroli, Villa Santo Stefano, Trivigliano
- Viterbo: Orte
- Ascoli Piceno: Ascoli Piceno, Castel di Lama, Offida
- Umbria: Terni

Regarding the earthquake in the L'Aquila Province, the relationship between the population and the institutions was particular and very interesting for its social process and social representations. During some interviews, people told me that they had informed the local and regional authorities about the little shocks before the big one, but they were told there was no reason to be anxious or nervous about them. The question here is not the polemic on this issue, because this is a sociological work, but I think it is important to take into consideration when thinking about the implications for the future relationship between administrations and their citizens.

The reconstruction phase in L'Aquila is in a latency period because of the trial and legislative questions that arose after this earthquake and the conditions in which people live: there has been a distance between the people and the institutions, with deep roots in the social process of crisis and disaster management. Furthermore, there is a visible lack of collaborative pattern and civil trust between the municipality and the citizens: these two elements seem to have put a stop to the reconstruction activities shared by the public administrations and the people living there.

5.4.1 *My Arrival in L'Aquila and Monticchio*

The first time I was in L'Aquila, I observed the mobility and a traffic jam along the only passable streets. I went downtown and saw something incredible. In the inner city of L'Aquila there was not a single building that was saved from the earthquake, and all the buildings had been shored up by firemen. Some edifices seem to be in the reconstruction phase, but most should probably be pulled down.

The loss of cultural heritage is felt deeply in the social and institutional life of the city. It is worth remembering that L'Aquila is the capital of the Abruzzo region, and all the administrative offices and public administration necessary for the city itself and the whole region are concentrated there.

Moreover, the traffic jam, one of the consequences of the social and lifestyle changes after the earthquake, is not the only thing I could see: for a sociologist, people are the principal subject, and there were many people there who attracted my attention. This was because of the personal and social conditions in which they currently lived: the sorrow and posttraumatic stress after the disaster can be recognized even without clinical analysis. People were disoriented, confused, and completely destroyed by the change of physical and spatial surroundings and landscapes.

The destruction of L'Aquila and its surroundings means the destruction of many communities, lives, and social ties. What it is more painful than all these dramatic experiences is the feeling of being in a ghost city: no people, no buildings, no services, no infrastructure, no shops. There I understood completely, for the first time in my life, what it means to lose everything and not have the possibility of coping with a disaster.

The military controls the center of L'Aquila, both for security reasons and for the safety of the people, but it is not a good image – think of your own city and the military on the street corners. We are right in the middle of a civil defense approach, but I believe people need hope and the possibility to go on. In my opinion, the situation requires the responsibility of making decisions and realizing them: safeguarding historical buildings and cultural heritage needs to be connected with the practical life of the people and the reconstruction of the city and its social life.

Monticchio was different: it is a little town and the people in the community are closer to one another, and new houses have been built by the state. The physical and human proximity made a difference, even if many things must still be reconstructed.

When I returned home, I thought that something should be done. I hope that this situation does not remain in this chronic manner for much longer.

Chapter 6
Civil Protection Voluntary Service: An Introduction to the Issue Through Interviews with Experts

Chapter 6 introduces and analyzes the collection of nine semistructured interviews with civil protection experts at local, provincial, and regional levels. These semistructured interviews were aimed at understanding the Civil Protection Voluntary Service during the past 60 years, its changes in organization, and its prosocial culture. I decided to focus attention on local, provincial, and regional levels because in these contexts the Civil Protection Voluntary Service has various and fundamental activities, competencies, roles, and skills.

After the presentation and analysis of the content from the interviews, useful features and dimensions emerged to orient the creation of an online questionnaire for all civil protection volunteers at a national level. In particular, these included Italian civil protection volunteers and their main motivations for becoming civil protection volunteers, the importance of the relationships among civil protection volunteers, the organization of civil protection voluntary associations, and volunteers' roles and competencies within disaster planning and management.

6.1 Introduction

Voluntary service in contemporary times has become an important issue within the context of civil society and its collaborative and participative pattern. Voluntary service, within all social fields, represents one of the highest indicators of democracy and active participation in one's own society. It is directly connected with solidarity among, altruism of, and help offered and received by people with different difficulties in their lives (Godbout 1992).

As mentioned earlier, in Italy the importance and competency of the Civil Protection Voluntary Service has been increasing, although sometimes a lack remains among some diverse levels of civil protection voluntary work. Civil protection voluntary work in Italy can be connected with the general system of voluntary work and is considered the third sector: "the development of the third sector in Italy

B. Lucini, *Disaster Resilience from a Sociological Perspective*, Humanitarian Solutions in the 21st Century, DOI 10.1007/978-3-319-04738-6_6,

goes back to the mid-1970s when the dyadic system, made up of the Market and the State, became obsolete, as it was no longer capable of satisfying all the needs and emerging instances of an evolving society" (Rapizza and Held 2006). According to this definition, civil protection voluntary work is also a component of the third sector; in particular, it is organized through diverse forms of organization such as local groups within the municipality, associations, and provincial and regional groups.

It is worth considering the language and cultural distinction of civil protection voluntary work or service that is connected to the community; rather than an unpaid apprenticeship, voluntary service is regarded as unpaid but requiring professional skills. In Italy, civil protection voluntary work is certainly like this; in this book, the phrase "voluntary service or work" is used because it underlines the connection to the community.

The analysis by Rapizza and Held (2006) recognizes the role of identification made possible by "the framework law on volunteering, Law No. 266/91 recognizes the social value and function of volunteering as an expression of participation, solidarity and pluralism. This law officially defined in 1991 the characteristics of voluntary organisations and the aspects that regulate the relationship between the voluntary organizations and the public administration, together with the juridical recognition of public entity partners."

Volunteering is not a new activity in Italy. It has been a force even in past eras, for example, during the 13th century, the Confraternite della Misericordia based in Toscana was created. Nevertheless, in this field evolution was continual and related to the historical period.

"During the 1970s, important welfare reforms took place, including Law No. 833/1978 Institution of National Health System which acknowledge the role of volunteering in art. 45" (Rapizza and Held 2006), but it was in the 1990s "that it brought big legislative changes regarding voluntary activity, from the Volunteering Framework Law 266/1991, defining the characteristics of voluntary organisation, to Law no. 383/2000 regulating social promotion organizations" (Rapizza and Held 2006).

As we will see in the next chapter, during this period civil protection volunteering also was implemented. In particular, with Law no. 225/1992 regarding the operative structures of the Italian civil protection system, voluntary organizations became a formal component of the Italian civil protection system. Law no. 194/2001 established the conditions by which they could be admitted to the regional civil protection voluntary register.

What changed during these years is the conception of the citizen as having an important role in the social and institutional life of her/his nation. In particular, there was an increased awareness of participation and collaboration in activities, which are based on solidarity and general prosocial attitudes.

The so-called welfare mix, a sort of cooperation between citizens and public institutions, was created: "there was also a significant change in the relationship between the State and the citizens, who were now capable of greater participation and organization in answering to the needs of society and dealing with issues of 'general interest', by operating directly on the territory" (Rapizza and Held 2006).

Civil protection voluntary work is identified as a fundamental component of the civil protection system, but the question is more complex. In particular, according to this general introduction to the voluntary work sector in Italy, the original idea of disaster resilience from a sociological perspective is based on a proposal to consider civil protection volunteers as key figures with a central role in ensuring an adequate response to a disaster and, more important, in preventive and preparedness planning. In fact, the relationship between civil protection volunteers and the population at risk or affected by a disaster should be carefully explored to understand its sociological implications and the influence during the impact of and the first response to the disaster (Norris and Kaniasty 1996). Some social behaviors such as altruism, solidarity, and prosocial action and assistance must be taken into account, as are competitive and conflict actions.

This argument started with some theoretical assumptions, which assumed the role of a theoretical background for this theme and, in particular, attention was focused on the research work done by Marta and Pozzi (2007) on the psychology of voluntary service. It would also present the main useful interpretative model for the area of civil protection voluntary service in Italy. On an empirical level, to deeply comprehend this peculiar relationship, semistructured interviews were conducted with nine experts from the Civil Protection Voluntary Service in Milan and in the Lombardia region.

- Male Civil Protection Voluntary Service expert and civil protection volunteer with more than 30 years of experience in this field
- Female president of an association within which the area of the Civil Protection Voluntary Service exists
- Male involved in the Civil Protection Voluntary Service in the Lombardia region
- Female 1 involved in the Civil Protection Voluntary Service in the Lombardia region
- Female 2 involved in the Civil Protection Voluntary Service in the Lombardia region
- Male 1 involved in the Civil Protection Voluntary Service in the province of Milan
- Male 2 involved in the Civil Protection Voluntary Service in the province of Milan
- Male involved in the Civil Protection Voluntary Service in the province of Brescia
- Male involved in the Civil Protection Voluntary Service in the municipality of Milan

These interviews were collected in the period between January and March 2011. The practical information gleaned from them was used to create the online questionnaire for civil protection volunteers. The original intent of the questionnaire was to virtually combine many opinions and experiences by civil protection volunteers, an action that could not possibly be done in another manner because of the organizational structure of the Civil Protection Voluntary Service in Italy, as previously explained.

6.2 Brief Overview of the Theoretical Background of the Civil Protection Voluntary Service

Studying the world of the Civil Protection Service in Italy is a difficult activity because of the organizational and structural characteristics of the service itself. As I said before, the main interpretative models for voluntary service according to Marta and Pozzi (2007) would be the following:

- Volunteer process model by Omoto and Snyder (1995)
- Role identity model of voluntarism by Callero and Piliavin (1987)
- Sustained voluntarism model by Penner (1998)
- The model proposed by Davis (2005)
- Integrative model for voluntarism process by Marta and Pozzi (2007)
- Three-stage model of volunteers' duration by Chacòn et al. (2006)
- A new model

The first model presented is based on the motivations that move people to become volunteers. The model is constructed through three phases: before the choice, experiences, and consequences, all at three different levels of analysis: individual, organizational, and social. The central questions in this theoretical model are the motivations and personal needs that cause people to choose the activity of voluntary service. Omoto and Snyder (1995) consider the personal disposition to help and prosocial attitudes as the basis for voluntary service. Moreover, voluntary service has the peculiarity of enhancing personal and professional capacity. The intentions to continue with voluntary activities is influenced by positive satisfaction and personal efficacy.

The second model, the role identity model of voluntarism by Callero and Piliavin (1987), is characterized by the situational elements and focuses less on the dispositional elements mentioned above. The roles played by volunteers is the fundamental element on which the model is based. Much attention is dedicated to the organizational aspects and their characteristics to enhance the voluntary service. A sense of belonging to the organization and the link between social role and social identity are the characteristics of this model. The assumption within this theory is that the role identity of the volunteer is connected with the actions done as volunteer, with less regard for the sense of belonging to the organizations or to the voluntary group.

The third model is the sustained voluntarism model by Penner (1998). It represents an integration of the two previous models. In particular, it is developed through a timeline; the first phase starts with dispositional attitudes and the decision to become a volunteer. The second phase is the real experience of voluntary service, followed by the construction of the role identity and maintenance of it over time.

The fourth model was elaborated by Davis (2005) and focuses on personal variables that influence voluntary activities. Personality is the key concept for this model related/linked to different phases of voluntary process listed previously.

The fifth model is the integrative model for voluntarism process by Marta and Pozzi (2007), and it arises from an integration of motivation oriented toward other people and satisfaction with and integration in the volunteer organization to which a person belonged. The research done by Marta and Pozzi seems to confirm the hypothesis that these two key elements influence and determine the role identity of volunteers.

The sixth model is the three-stage model of volunteers' duration by Chacòn et al. (2006). It is based on the study of the duration of voluntary activities. Accordingly, they found that three stages, or times, predict duration: early satisfaction, organizational involvement at the mid-term, and role identity over the long-term.

Each model presented so far has elaborated the voluntary process in a specific area of research and has taken into account a specific population for the study. The seventh model is a new one. Marta and Pozzi (2007) tried to systematize the previous models into four macro categories: prosocial personality, motivations, identity, and culture organization.

The interviews with the experts in the Civil Protection Voluntary Service, mentioned earlier, and the online questionnaire for all civil protection volunteers (Chap. 7) at national, regional, provincial and local levels were understood and created according to this theoretical introduction.

6.3 Interviews with Experts in Civil Protection Voluntary Service

After taking into account the cited interpretative models of voluntary process (Omoto and Malsch 2005), and considering interesting assumptions about roles and social identities within a sociological discussion of volunteerism actions, the following outline for the interviews with experts was created, with the specific aim of understanding better the roles and the organization of the civil protection service. Particular attention focused on sociological implications within role identity, sense of community, and sense of belonging and the complex personalities of volunteers who were involved in civil protection.

The outline for the interviews comprised an introduction, a first part focusing on voluntary service within civil protection, a second part asking about the relationships between volunteers and civil protection associations, a third part looking at relationships between civil protection volunteers and the population affected by critical events, and a conclusion.

It started with an introduction to the research and the general question, "Who is the civil protection volunteer, for you?" The aim of this question was to explore the cognitive images and perceptions of volunteers in general as understood by experts in the Civil Protection Voluntary Service. Different and interesting answers were collected, focusing three main themes.

Availability of time: "The volunteer is a person who dedicates free time for a project, an idea that was interesting. I said 'free time' because it is time one finds and takes from the family. . . (male CPVS expert). Another expert noted that "the volunteer is a person who can give time; I do not talk about free time because many people work, but those who can give time to relief aid, organization, and orientation aids to the population" (female 2, Lombardia region). Time is also connected with passion, and this feeling is basilar to those who do voluntary activities: "A person who makes free time to dedicate her/himself to something in which they believe and have passion, because now, with the actual system, if you have no passion, it is difficult to do voluntary service because it is almost a kind of second job if you do it conscientiously and with intensity" (Male 1, province of Milan).

To gift something: "A volunteer is a person who feels the need to gift something of her/himself, not only listening and empathy but also in terms of time and over and above the technical competencies" (Male, province of Brescia).

At an institutional level, *seeing the volunteer as a citizen*: "The volunteer is a citizen, she/he learns to be a citizen using her/his desire, at the beginning, that does not depend on external situations, but has its origins in an internal maturity, so a willingness that does not mean wishing to do many things or any emotional feeling, but a desire to be useful, enhancing the circles in which she/he lives and for this reason enhancing her/himself, so the volunteer is a person who works on his/her own ideas and is less egoistic" (female president of association). Another expert also noted that "The volunteer is a citizen who has the will to gift her/himself to another person or other people who have problems, so she/he is a person who has the desire to dedicate her/himself to the others" (male, municipality of Milan). The institutional level is also represented by the way the Civil Protection Service is organized in a hierarchical model: "It does this within a context that functions in a hierarchical model" (male, province of Brescia).

Therefore, the image of the volunteer according to a general area of interest is characterized by three levels of perception:

1. To have time available seems to be an organizational and structural aspect for identifying volunteers and defining their work.
2. On a personal and individual level, having a desire to gift time, help, and support to people living in difficult conditions and who have problems.
3. The volunteer as a citizen means the institutional participation of volunteers within the civil society. This point is particularly interesting regarding the philosophical and practical implications to the civil society system as presented by Margalit (1998) and his concept of a decent society.

Points 1 and 2 also have importance regarding the motivations that move people to make the decision to become a volunteer.

Here, the specific aim is to understand whether there is a discrepancy between the image of the volunteer in general and civil protection volunteers in particular. For this reason, the civil protection experts were asked to specify, if possible, what kind of person volunteers: “Can you define the typical person who becomes a civil protection volunteer?”

In this context there is always the presence of an institution; the question focused on the fact that “the civil protection volunteer is a person who came into being in the voluntary service world at the beginning of the 1980s and precisely because she/he was a public assistance volunteer for civil protection, without hav[ing] knowledge of civil protection, and this is demonstrated by the law 225/1992” (male CPVS expert).

The institutional level is also represented by the “question of organization, without structure; we have a regulation, it is a new regulation that substitutes the older and it gives the general norms that, in my opinion, need to be clearly fixed at local and regional levels in the orientation of Augustus method” (female 2, Lombardia region). In this context, the issue of available time arose as part of the definition of the civil protection volunteer: “the civil protection volunteer is always available . . . and then she/he dedicates her/his time not only to help people, but also to prevent the damage which can occur in an emergency” (female 1, Lombardia region). Time is also connected “in our specific case because you are aware that you do not work every day, but you can work only once a year, but perhaps that time you work for 3 months and in difficult circumstances, where people have lost every landmark and so you are the landmark for those people” (male, municipality of Milan).

A specific distinction results from the difference between time of emergency and time of no emergency. “Civil Protection Voluntary Services, in the past, has been collocated at the time of the emergency, so it has been perceived as only involved in an emergency. Fortunately, now it has been understood that it can be useful in everyday life and also for prevention and planning, and in many other important daily activities, thinking, for example, of a qualified volunteer, it is right to have unskilled labor, but if I need added value, I must go through education, training and these things need a lot of time” (male CPVS expert).

Another aspect involved is the competencies and work of the Civil Protection Voluntary Service: “the world of civil protection is an exclusively technical world, so at the base there should be a personal interest” (male 1, province of Milan). The image of the civil protection volunteer is always defined in a positive way: “in my opinion they are people with a huge sense of generosity and responsibility” (female president of association).

Differences have been noted according to the question of time in terms of continuity of service, confronting other kinds of voluntary service, and the emergency context of the job: “there are the differences in terms of continuity” (male, province of Brescia). Also, “the meeting with the others . . . instead becomes occasional or, for some kind of activities, there is no meeting with the others because, if you work at a specific emergency, there is a meeting not only with your colleagues or institutions but also with the environment” (male, province of Brescia).

The major differences between voluntary service in other areas and the Civil Protection Voluntary Service can be summarized according to the following points:

- The type of timeline along which the activities of volunteers take place is continuous versus occasional.
- Meeting with people who are in difficult situations or have many problems is different according to the quality of the meeting itself, the needs of the people, the context, and the duration of the voluntary activities.
- In general the imagine of civil protection volunteers is correlated to some positive attitudes such as generosity, responsibility, help offered, solidarity, collaboration, altruism, prosocial behaviour, and trust. This consideration has helped to focus attention on the important motivations behind becoming a civil protection volunteer and in the creation of the online questionnaire dedicated to them.

6.4 Why Become a Civil Protection Volunteer?

Taking into consideration the interpretative model of volunteerism and, above all, motivations that are the basis for the choice to become a civil protection volunteer, this dimension was explored with the previous civil protection experts to orient the construction of the online questionnaire dedicated to civil protection volunteers. This process was helped by the use of the Voluntary Function Inventory, a scale of 30 items exploring 6 dimensions of motivation, with responses of agree or not agree: value motivation, knowledge, career, social, protection, self-enhancement. The value of motivation is considered other-oriented, whereas the others are self-oriented.

In particular, the following question was asked of the experts: "According to you, what are the main motivations for becoming a civil protection volunteer?" Some interesting answers must be highlighted.

The issue of available time is presented here as a motivation to become a civil protection volunteer: "a civil protection volunteer is interested because she/he has a lot of free time and she/he wants to do something useful" (female 2, Lombardia region).

Motivations also are correlated with social attitudes such as help and solidarity. "after 45 years of civil protection voluntary service, I can say that, if I weigh up successes and failures, I am not interested in how many people I has assisted, I don't have these kind of statistics, perhaps it is more about what I have received than [what] I have given" (male CPVS expert). The same expert also noted that, "in the end all people have need of others, it is not because I give to others that makes me better than the others."

Another interesting issue about motivations for choosing civil protection voluntary service is that of becoming a volunteer versus being born a volunteer. It is a basilar issue because it arises from a psychological and sociological background coming from culture, family, socialization process, personal attitudes. and feelings. "Motivation belongs to the single person, what I have learned, when I was young, one time at a conference they asked me, 'Do you become or were you born as a volunteer?' I have contested this sentence, because it is true that you become volunteer, you have courses in the area you have chosen, but a volunteer is born if, in her/his family, there is a culture that fostered the desire to be a volunteer, to dedicate to others" (male CPVS expert). The importance in the influence of this expert's choice to volunteer, which is attributed to the family within which he grew up and his intergenerational background, is interesting.

Again, motivations remain deeply personal and individual: "in my opinion you always start with this, not knowing the world of voluntary service personally, you join one group or another and then you find yourself a volunteer and in the end you learn things and you are dedicated to others, therefore always with a positive attitude, an attitude of responsibility. What is missing is an awareness that the volunteer is a person with a big inner world, which you must understand and that, in case of necessity, in case of external pressure, you can use to remain stable and really useful" (female president of association). The inner world seems be a peculiar attribution for the voluntary personality, not only at a personal and individual level but also in a case of emergency; it is considered a resource for the volunteer and, as a consequence, for the people helped by her/him.

Many experts said that motivations are a personal issue: "motivations are so subjective that it is not possible to standardize [them] . . .perhaps they are influenced by their culture (male 1, province of Milan). Another expert noted that, "they are strong motivations that are obviously oriented according to their own experience and their own culture and preparedness" (male, Lombardia region). The interview with this expert also underlined the difficulty in exploring and comprehending a topic such as motivation.

It seems true that a sort of polarity exists that makes the distinction between self-oriented motivations and other-oriented motivations possible, both those in the field of civil protection voluntary service as well those presented by the previous cited Voluntary Function Inventory. Other-oriented motivations are constituted by "solidarity and offered help to the others" (female 1, Lombardia region).

One of the most interesting motivations for becoming a civil protection volunteer, as given by one of the experts, is correlated with the social role of the volunteer and the channel of socialization of this activity:

> it could also be the publicity, we have seen in these last few years publicity for national civil protection, but also regional, municipality, or provinces, which has driven the recruitment of new volunteers, so a sort of publicity to find volunteers makes a person curious if she/he has this spirit or maybe only make an approach to understand how it is. . . . On one hand this communicative method drives the person who has the direct mental connection to approach, on the other hand she/he can have the spirit to do it, not always in a constant way, so she/he must choose to volunteer in a field that doesn't bind her/him because, for example, in the socio-health area, being a member of the ambulance service or [working at night] makes it harder. (Male, municipality of Milan)

There arises the point that there is an institutional lack of understanding of civil protection voluntary service as a continuous activity for a whole year and not only in cases of emergency, and for its impact period.

Someone else remembered that civil protection volunteers and the institutions that aim to organize the civil protection system should always be involved in different kinds of activities and during all theoretical phases of a disaster. For example, with regard to the mitigation and preventive and preparedness phases, they consider these times as moments of inactivity or breaks that makes the voluntary service "simpler and not so binding," a misinterpretation that should be regularized at a cultural and organizational level.

6.5 Prosocial Attitudes and Their Role Within the Activities of the Civil Protection Voluntary Service

We have seen the main motivations represented by a personal "spirit" to dedicate oneself to others and attitudes such as solidarity, collaboration, altruism, prosociality, and trust. For this reason it is interesting to explore the role of these social attitudes within the activities of the Civil Protection Voluntary Service. The experts were asked: "Which role did you assume – attitudes such as solidarity, collaboration, altruism, prosociality, and trust – within the activities of civil protection voluntary service?"

The first aspect is the recognition of volunteers and their social attitudes as basilar elements to volunteerism.

In my opinion they are the base, that is, a person does not work on this feeling, on the availability and the growing up of availability; it is clear that, when a person is in different situations of life, which can be a difficult personal situation, or can also be a simple engagement or a different job, that you can find in a normal path of life, she/he will leave the voluntary service because she/he will consider it as something added that she/he can renounce and now it is the voluntary service, but also it can be many other associations, e.g., scouting; however, they have a small percentage of adults involved because people leave. (Female president of association)

The male CVS expert stated that, "it is a great number of people who are dedicated to helping others, many of them have high capabilities, they are always ready to play their role, to experience and grow, and then they are part of the operative system and they have the skills to be useful in emergencies." The concepts highlighted here are very interesting in terms of the maintenance of a volunteer's commitment. In fact:

> the maintenance of voluntary activity from when a person is young means that, when they encounter their first difficulties, the first changes in life, the person leaves. For this reason, the volunteer needs support; it is clear that the way of approach by the voluntary service organization must change, but to do this it must mature, it should not hold the volunteer back, otherwise they don't grow as a person and then the voluntary service has this capacity of uniting people with high human qualities, that is, the friendship that grows through the voluntary service, it is a lasting friendship, it is not circumstantial. (Female president of association)

Another core issue is represented by personal and individual predisposition: "it is a subjective question . . . interests are cultivated with time so they grow with time . . . if, in a family, there is a civil protection culture, then the children are introduced to this world, perhaps they choose other forms of voluntary service" (male 1, province of Milan).

As seen here, time has an important role that should be taken into consideration within the voluntary service, and specifically in the Civil Protection Voluntary Service, because of its three fundamental dimensions:

- Time as generational time: a reflection on the example given by the family to become a volunteer and in a context of intergenerational exchange, even if, for this question, one should not forget the role of culture and its practical influences.
- Time as historical and personal conditions: before this, the availability of time to become a volunteer has been correlated with older people and the period of retirement, with the assumption that time was more available than during other phases of one's life. It is interesting that, for this purpose, time is considered in terms of age: "I have observed that, for young people, only those who are more interested or where it is prearranged approach [to voluntary service], but we can say that, probably, mentally, the information does not arrive in the right way to young people and those who are considering it [are] already oriented to see the world as "I want to help"; that is, there is not, perhaps, proper preparation; that is, perhaps it is better, really, to start with the schools to give these inputs, to allow comprehension of the importance of giving" (female 2, Lombardia region).
- Time in terms of emergency or nonemergency and within the context of the Civil Protection Voluntary Service: it is fundamental for the analysis of the motivations for becoming a civil protection volunteer:

> If you do not consider the social needs, you cannot not even give norm to behaviors or orient behaviors during the emergency, where you are asked, in a very short time, to respond to real needs where they have an urgency. Another question instead is planning an event, . . . that is, answering [a] different need, but it is always a social need, so they are different things, one you can plan, even if not fully, because you cannot plan everything, but you can plan many things; instead first you must plan in the time of no emergency, trying to approach the emergency scenario in which you could work in the best way possible, but also the unforeseeable things are very possible, that is, in the sense that, although you have all the norms to face, there will be things which you have absolutely not evaluated, because this is the way it is, all the time something unexpected happens, it is a training experience, if you also have briefing and debriefing, you can understand what has failed and what can be improved" (female 2, Lombardia region).

The time of emergency is a "special" time and it needs particular attention to understand the behaviors of civil protection volunteers during this period: "Then when you are in emergency you have a double channel: one is demonstrating that you know how to do something, perhaps little things, but it must be demonstrated to the leaders . . . that I am able to do this is the first thing; according to me. The second more important thing is that what moves people to do this is altruism, the desire to help people, to receive a smile and make people feel good, including in a moment when she/he has lost everything, thinking, for example, of Abruzzo, Haiti, Sri Lanka" (male, municipality of Milan).

This basilar attitude of altruism remains: "volunteers have a predisposition to help the others primarily from the human aspect, i.e., to give help in case of necessity; according to me this is the main motivation" (female 1, Lombardia region). Civil protection volunteers are represented as "people who work very hard and do not only start at 7 a.m. and end at midnight, they sleep very little, with the aim of giving a smile to another person" (male, municipality of Milan).

Prosocial attitudes have a fundamental role within the whole Civil Protection Voluntary Service because they are the base upon which the activities of voluntarism are constructed. Then they influence the choice to become a volunteer of a civil protection area and orient future actions in this specific field.

6.6 The Civil Protection Voluntary Service in the Regions of Italy

Regarding the general aim of this research and the specific understanding of civil protection volunteers and their possible role in disaster resilience at different levels (local, provincial, regional, and national), it was necessary to explore the existence of differences in this volunteerism field throughout the regions of Italy and, in particular, the regions in which three earthquakes occurred: Umbria and Marche in 1997, Molise in 2002, and Abruzzo in 2009.

Therefore, the civil protection experts were asked: "Are there any peculiarities and/or differences participating in civil protection volunteer services between different regions of Italy and, more specifically, between Umbria, Marche, Molise, and Abruzzo?"

Some experts said that they did not know exactly whether there are any profound differences among regions themselves of Italy, and probably it is due to the local boundaries and competition between regions that are always present in this field. In fact, the civil protection system in Italy often is seen as a specific area that allows diverse people to show their value and their abilities; this goes beyond the simple sense of belonging to an institution: "it is the impression that if some people have personal deficiencies, they would be able to develop themselves, wear the uniform and believe in themselves – to be someone" (male CPVS expert). This expert also stated that "the uniform is a box, what it contains makes the difference. We can understand this [by] observing the volunteers in the last few emergencies, and it is deplored that, during the first day of the emergency, there are television crews and the mass media on site with volunteers represented by their new uniforms, not just clean but new, and this is strange thinking to be a volunteer is to be humble and giving of her/his availability."

This argument points out the question of ethics in disaster research within the specific area of the Civil Protection Voluntary Service and, in general, people giving relief aid. In spite of the earlier comments, some people referred to differences between the regions regarding the Civil Protection Voluntary Service and not between volunteers themselves:

> Yes, there are many differences because we have without doubt an excellence, and this is without trying to exploit or make some racial comment on the difference between the North and the South. There is obviously a culture of voluntary service. I come from a health voluntary service which I started doing when I was 18 years old. It was their 60th anniversary of Public Assistance, in 1966 there were not so many people in public assistance, but you can understand that voluntary service was common only as far as Tuscany, we know that Tuscany is the center of voluntary service, the place where the Confraternite della Misericodia was started in the 1200s. Then the culture of voluntary service extended as far as South Italy, there are also some excellent services in the South, they are becoming the same as in the North. . . .
>
> This is also because in our times there wasn't a culture for these associations, so I and my friends, all with the same thought to do something, something to help others, it is not something that satisfies myself, my need, because it's not voluntary service; the aim is to solve the need of another person, to help her/him in her/his moment of need and within an association.
>
> In the last few years, the civil protection area has been developed by local groups which depend on the mayor, and so there is no expression of association experience, that is completely another subject. I would not say that within the local group there aren't people having and feeling this need for voluntary service in the same way as an association because, in the end, the association is the thing that gives you the desire to believe and fight for what you have created and that you want to grow. . . . Unfortunately I must say that the association service is dying, the State forgets those who want to help other people, I say that in a general sense and not only for civil protection, thinking for a while of those who work in hospitals, with cancer patients, children, youths, the elderly, so the voluntary service makes a less visible splash than those who wear the coloured uniform and who are more visible on the television" (male CPVS expert).

The issue of North and South Italy is an old one, and in the voluntary service there is the presence of differences depending on the place in Italy in which the activities have taken place: "in the North/central North there is a voluntary service that would be specialist, it would be as if it were specialist. . . . In some regions of the central South, perhaps, it is a different thing because of a sense of spirit that may be more than in the North; unfortunately there are [fewer] institutions and agencies which believe in the voluntarism activity than in the central North" (male, Lombardia region).

Attention should be focused on the following relevant issues:

- The image of the Civil Protection Voluntary Service and the sense of belonging to an institution with the aim of helping people in case of need, specifically regarding to natural or technological disasters
- The difference in the historical process of voluntary service and the territorial differences among the regions in Italy, in particular North and South Italy, which present a peculiar development process because of the their cultural, political, and institutional variables
- Motivations, which are multidimensional issues and that, as previously explained, are expressed as personal and individual attitudes

Differences also are present not only at a cultural or institutional level but also according to the characteristics of the people involved as civil protection volunteers:

> I have noticed a unique difference, that I have directly observed concerning the Abruzzo and Lombardia regions. In Abruzzo I met many volunteers, aged 27, 30 years old, whereas many volunteers who came together in the Lombardia region are older than that and you may have a volunteer who is 50 years old she/he and is considered to be young. This is the difference at a social level because the voluntary system is perceived as an activity to do during one's free time, but our voluntary service, that we propose, is a voluntary service where the young can be involved in society and so becom[e] aware citizens, conscious and useful to the world that surrounds them; for this our volunteers have a medium age which is very low, the majority are from 18 to 30 years old. It is clear that the president is older than the others, but this tends to be the limit for the volunteers" (female president of association).

The principle differences that are peculiar to the Civil Protection Voluntary Service in Italy are summarized as follows:

- Territorial differences linked with the institutional and cultural framework within which they should take place
- Personal differences of age, linked with the individual characteristics of volunteers belonging to civil protection volunteer groups and the territorial gap
- Differences linked with specific culture and the training experience of civil protection volunteers

The following analysis is oriented on the second part of the interview, which focused on the relationship between volunteers and civil protection associations. In particular, it was considered that this relationship is basilar and fundamental to understanding the culture of the Civil Protection Voluntary Service and the organization of activities in times of emergency or no emergency.

6.7 Relationships and Interactions Between Civil Protection Volunteers

According to the aim of exploring the social relationships of civil protection volunteers, to understand how the online questionnaire was used at national level better and believing in its benefit to the theoretical framework of professional resilience, the following questions were of the experts.

1. According to you, which characteristics mark the interactions between volunteers and your own association with particular reference to the Umbria and Marche (1997), Molise (2002), and Abruzzo (2009) earthquakes?
2. How, do you believe, have the volunteers committed to the same group interacted in the Umbria and Marche (1997), Molise (2002), and Abruzzo (2009) earthquakes?

3. Which roles did you assume, according to you, e.g., attitudes such as solidarity, collaboration, and trust among volunteers committed to the same group, in the Umbria and Marche (1997), Molise (2002), Abruzzo (2009) earthquakes?

The first question focuses on the relationship between the civil protection volunteer and her/his own association or municipality group of civil protection to explore and understand dynamics such as leadership, organization, and a sense of belonging. Many interesting points arose.

Many interesting points have been found.

The relationship between volunteers and her/his association are not always idyllic. "Taking into consideration that volunteers or those who represent them are men and, according to me, for this reason there are human weakness[es], with values and faults like everywhere. All people are [like this], so the relationship between volunteers and associations are not always idyllic, also because the volunteer, after a while, feels herself/himself responsible . . . and the phenomena of bullying is very concealed; a person can say 'I have been here for a long time and instead you have just arrived'" (female 1, Lombardia region). This underlines the hierarchical organization and logic that sometimes exist in the civil protection voluntary association or local group.

The relationship is also dependent upon the people who constitute the organizations:

> it depends, depends on the type of organization and on the way in which the people are organized. It is dependent on the lead person, also at a provincial level, but also on the funding which is set aside for civil protection activities by different structures such as the municipality, province, region and the training activities that are proposed. . . . That is the really important thing; sometimes volunteers understand that civil protection activity works according to a hierarchical logic more than the leader does, they have a very clear idea about this structure, even, sometimes, they rise up against the leader . . ." (female 2, Lombardia region).

In addition to this position, there is another point of view that concentrates on the positive relationship between civil protection volunteers and her/his association: "In my opinion the civil protection volunteer must feel good with other people with [whom] they share the activities, so they must have a strong tie with others . . ., it is important to work together with other organizations because sharing activities are possible, sharing your opinion with others, and there is the creation of a network among different members, otherwise they have the orientation to be isolated. . ." (male, province of Brescia).

Another interesting observation follows:

> In our association there are no differences, this situation exists because of the people within it, there is no division, there is no hierarchical logic, there is a lead person, but it is a natural organization based on experiences because experience is important and groups should be led by a person with experience in this field. But also the last person can do experience and there is a sort of changeover among generations done by simplicity and availability . . . everyone has her/his role, a little or large responsibility, no activity is paid, but our voluntary service is an authentic voluntary service; everyone gives what she/he wants and assumes responsibilities according to their beliefs and their choices, that is better than being

forced to do it. Hence here, in our association, there is no difference and it is not only the civil protection voluntary service, because there are also social, cultural, and environmental fields, but it is all an authentic voluntary service" (female president of association).

Other points of view regarding this peculiar relationship are determined by juridical and structural opinions. "Yes, also the voluntary service is constituted by the regional register; in some regions the register exists because there is a law, but the law is not enough because it also has to work accounting for the volunteers and their needs. It is not possible to consider it just because there is a law" (male, Lombardia region).

The aspect of participation within the institutional agencies seems to be characteristic of the Civil Protection Voluntary Service:

It is dependent on the organization of the municipality, the volunteer should be part of a system and not feel used or utilized. For this reason we use the word *engage*, . . . we have placed volunteers within the system, we are not the only municipality which proposes courses or training experiences . . . but we have given them a place, a specific room for their activities, where they can meet together as an association, because we should guarantee a different, more flexible way of thinking; so proposals should also come from the volunteers, otherwise they are passive, because it seems that we impose all things but it is not so. For this reason a coordination plan exists . . . the relationship must be two-sided or bidirectional" (male, municipality of Milan).

These interviews highlighted an important point – that is, the ambivalent relationship existing between civil protection volunteers and their association of voluntary groups – for the construction of the online questionnaire. One possible initial consideration is the difference between the structure of the local group within the municipality system as well as provincial and regional groups and the Civil Protection Voluntary Service organized as an association. It is not a juridical diversification, but it involves aspects such as organization, structure, role, and culture.

The second issue concentrates on the interaction between volunteers belonging to the same group (local groups, associations, etc.): "How, do you believe, have the volunteers committed to the same group interacted in the Umbria and Marche (1997), Molise (2002), and Abruzzo (2009) earthquakes?"

"Sometimes there is collaboration but also competition, in my opinion. In Abruzzo I observed that there definitely was collaboration, because without it there wouldn't have been the possibility to do anything; all that has been done, is because there was collaboration. . ., but it is clear among volunteers, they desire someone to tell them that they are good, they value this, and for this reason we said this to all volunteers; if not, maybe there is even a form of competition between them" (female 2, Lombardia region).

Collaboration and sharing values and objectives are important factors within a "healthy" association: "If the association is a 'healthy' association it gives a culture, a good collaboration means that all people think in the same way. It is important not to quarrel but to discuss about something we do not share, listen to another point of view, and do the best that we can do. . ., and I must do it in the best way possible, because the others expect that I do that" (male CPVS expert).

We have already seen the importance of emergency time and nonemergency time. Responses to questions about this issue underline the importance of this distinction.

> You need to distinguish the voluntary service activities in a time of emergency or in a time of peace . . . during an emergency, the activity of the voluntary service is hardly ever conflicting . . . because the mechanisms which characterized the intervention overcome the divisions. . . . In a time of peace, everywhere, some barriers still exist, from North to South, linked to competition among the different organizations of the Civil Protection Voluntary Service; in a time of peace, both now and in the future, that each service thinks it has the best practices in terms of organization and they would prefer that someone impose the standard or the law, and in my opinion it is wrong because it is from a low level that I construct something to propose at an institutional level" (male, Lombardia region).

Related to this, another expert stated: "In an emergency there is complete collaboration . . . to help people that need it, so everyone works in the same direction, and this is the strength of the Civil Protection Voluntary Service. When we are in ordinary times there is 'good' rivalry; it is the good rivalry that is also present within institutional agencies; instead it becomes self-defeating when you use it to underline your power" (male, municipality of Milan).

Conflicting elements seem to be present and "they bring people to breaking point and also people leave, volunteers who leave the world of voluntary service, but also the dynamics must be of mutual collaboration, and we should distinguish between local groups and associations of the Civil Protection Voluntary Service because the motivations will also be different. . ." (male, province of Brescia).

It should be made explicit that the ambivalence of feelings characterizing the interactions between volunteers cannot always be linked to the three specific Italian earthquakes because of the different participation of the experts interviewed during the earthquakes. However, positive feelings seem to be the basis of the voluntary service experience: "I can speak about my own association and the friendship is the basis for all . . . the friendly tie is very strong and I know I can count on them and the same is for them with me . . . it is an open friendship that receives and offers help to each other . . . there is this effort to create an emphatic relationship with others . . . a friendship with high values, constituted by total and almost complete trust" (female president of association).

Referring to the Abruzzo earthquake and coming back to the specificity of the three fields chosen for this analysis, one expert noted that, "the positivity of this earthquake [Abruzzo, 2009], if I may say so, is that the local voluntary service association have found that they are not alone. . . .The awareness of being in a group with many people is a resource, because a resource in a context such as L'Aquila, that I hope comes never again, the assistance in this way is dangerous that is 9, 8, 7 months in a civil protection camp to substitute the authority, this have permit to the provinces as Milan, to be present in a continuous way and this is a resource" (male 2, province of Milan).

Related to this issue of authority and the role of voluntary service, the third question was about the role of prosocial attitudes during the three Italian earthquakes: "Which roles did you assume, according to you, e.g., attitudes such as solidarity, collaboration, and trust among volunteers committed to the same group in the Umbria and Marche (1997), Molise (2002), and Abruzzo (2009) earthquakes?"

Interesting perspectives arose from this analysis, and they are concentrated on the different roles of prosocial attitudes; these are sometimes ambivalent, such as the relationship between civil protection volunteers and her/his associations, and assumed by the civil protection volunteers, specifically during an emergency. Some experts recognize that:

> there is a technical role, that is, the professionalism acquired by training, . . . and in our nation there are no serious guidelines or center dedicated to training in the civil protection field. . . . Certainly there are some lead regions such as the Lombardia region that has a regional school of civil protection; other examples are Venezia, Piemonte, . . . but not all agencies have continuity, their own philosophy for training or about the needs of and activities required by the volunteers, . . . and then it is clear that they have demonstrated they can be useful when, in the past, they were excluded. . . . The volunteers have enormous value. . ., they have demonstrated their indispensability. . . . Today they are also involved in the field of prevision and prevention, . . . if we take into consideration the evolution of civil protection activities the Umbria earthquake was the first time functions of support were activated" (male CPVS expert).

In this context, ambivalence and the complexity of the issue are determined by two different roles that civil protection volunteers assume. "There are a number of volunteers who are not in direct contact with the population. . ., but the volunteer does these activities, that means they are not in directly contact with the population, so there is a sort of hidden work that the general population may not always see, . . . because a volunteer could also be this, that is not only evident" (female 1, Lombardia region).

In spite of this vision, other experts believe that there is also direct contact with the population and that this is an important element during voluntary service:

> There is also direct contact with the population . . . and ties with the population, especially during the emergency, have been created unintentionally, where the activity of volunteer isn't specialized for the needs of population in that specific moment . . . and, so, a tie of sharing of this situation has been created . . . that must be separated from the general experience in that context; one must not be too involved, emotionally, to become occupied with a problem and make it yours with temporary solutions, but it is a problem of all people and you try to solve it as general problem" (male, Lombardia region).

Moreover, this contact with the population affected by an earthquake remains after a long period: ". . .we have worked as volunteers in contact with the population and we returned after that, during moments when people felt abandoned and alone. . . .[The] L'Aquila earthquake was different because there we were volunteers but also earthquake victims and this was a double role . . . the volunteers were the population . . . it was a wonderful training experience, these people with their own troubles, anyway they gave comfort and they have managed the camp for 8 months" (female president of association).

Even if there is ambivalence that seems to characterize the Civil Protection Voluntary Service, prosocial attitudes can be considered as the basis upon which it is possible to construct the real experience of voluntary service.

6.8 Relationship Between Civil Protection Volunteers and the Population Affected by Critical Events

The third part of the interview focused on the relationship between the civil protection volunteers and the population affected by critical events. The experts were asked the following questions:

1. Who, for the population, is the civil protection volunteer?
2. Which kind of relationships were there between the volunteers and the population in the Umbria and Marche (1997), Molise (2002), and the Abruzzo (2009) earthquakes?

The first question highlights an interesting view according to paradigm of reflexivity, which seems to be the new approach of sociological theory in the past 30 years.

The following was the most interesting answer to the first question listed above: "The population itself, because who can be a better rescuer than her/himself? Then, without doubt, we have need of others . . . the population itself always has a good view of voluntary service, . . . the uniform is well known because everyone has her/his own uniform and it is right that everyone who works in that sector can be identified and I know to whom I should go when I have a need" (male CPVS expert).

Another expert noted that, "the population identified the volunteers because they could see them more than they did with the institutions themselves . . . from the point of view of prevention it is right, but with a little distance, and this is has happened in some [southern] regions; there is also sort of cultural differences or particular cases within which the voluntary service cannot be not activated for specific civil protection activities" (male, Lombardia region).

Some aspects of this definition are linked with social and personal data – for example, age: "Consider that the civil protection volunteer is an old volunteer or, to put it better, there are [fewer] young people, there are few youths" (female 1, Lombardia region).

Another aspect is connected with the nationality of the civil protection volunteer: "Italian people have the ability to be flexible with procedures, so, she/he can improvise during the unexpected event. Referring to this approach I think the Italian people are not ready for this crisis management, there is the view that if something has happened, someone will take care of me" (male, municipality of Milan). However, on the other side, this expert also states that, "the citizen must take an active part within the system; she/he cannot stand alone, so the relationship depends on which region in which we are. In the North it is simpler and from the center South it is more difficult as an approach."

The commitment of the civil protection volunteer toward many activities that sometimes are not strictly related to civil protection activities can create confusion among the population and difficulty during the period of emergency management. "In my opinion the population is confused . . . because of the fact of the division in roles, because it is true that the local voluntary service could do diverse activities . . .

there is no clear idea about the voluntary service from the citizen, excluding the fire volunteers or the people involved in health care" (female 2, Lombardia region).

Experts noted positive and negative definitions concerning the figure of the civil protection volunteer: "They are well thought of, because if [they are] available and work in a good way they are well regarded. There have also been negative experiences, but they were the as for the last one, where the actions extended over a long period not only for the emergency, but there has been the creation of particular routines, so the population was also tired of everything" (male, province of Brescia). A positive definition also is represented by the following quote: "In our experience the volunteer is an angel, I do not have other experiences in other camps. . ., but I have seen a valued citizen, really valued . . . and it is difficult to explain, but they were valued" (female president of association).

According to the former quote, sometimes volunteers felt distanced from the population: "here you are the guests" (male 1, province of Milan). Also, referring to the L'Aquila earthquake, "the people who listen are emotionally involved . . . without receiving answers, and this is cannot come from the volunteer, but it must be an institutional response" (male 2, province of Milan).

The figure of the civil protection volunteer is, as seen before, ambivalent, and this is due to the particular role that is typical for this activity; it is also because of the institutional and administrative confusion that does not permit a clear understanding of the role and the activities that are owned by the civil protection volunteer.

6.9 Relationship Between Civil Protection Volunteers and the Population in the Last Three Earthquakes in Italy

The other fundamental question to try to understand the world of the Civil Protection Voluntary Service and its institutional role for the population was explored by the following question: "Which kind of relationships were there between the volunteers and the population in the Umbria and Marche (1997), Molise (2002), and Abruzzo (2009) earthquakes?" In this context, the earlier questions is valid. Because of their different experiences, roles, and professional positions, not all experts are able to completely answer this questions; however, some interesting reflections arose, mostly regarding the Abruzzo and L'Aquila earthquakes.

Different and negative behaviors were present during the L'Aquila earthquake.

> L'Aquila has had some problems because the relationship between the civil protection volunteers and the population sometimes has been a sort of affective-destructive attachment. There were three types of behavior: one person said I am here to help you, relax . . . you are my guest; there is, instead, the behavior of a person who identifies her/himself in that situation and then there is the behavior, perhaps from the majority of people, that they have the right to understand what their activity is; that was a moment of particular attention to the people and they supplanted the State for a period during which the State could not act" (male 2, province of Milan).

Other problems were noticed during the same earthquake:

> Yes, there were some cases, some little problems . . . I can say that when I was asked help by some people, for some jobs, . . . a few people accepted that it was more comfortable to be served by others . . . in fact, a few people collaborated with our camp, instead, I heard that in the other camp, Monticchio, there were people coming from the same community and this seemed a camp where people were in agreement and, in fact, they were involved in some activities of the camp itself, I can say they actively participated in the life of the camp" (female 1, Lombardia region).

Another critical situation, in addition to the minimal participation and collaboration from the population, was the sharing of public spaces and for a long period: "it was life in common, the period was so long within the same camp" (male 1, province of Milan).

Conflicting behaviours, as also depicted in the literature about the sociology of disasters (Clausen et al. 1978), have always been present:

> Hostilities can be created; don't forget that people affected by an event in that moment are not concerned about social relationships; on the contrary, they have needs and necessities. . . . It is clear that in this moment you need to interact with these people with much humbleness and understand their needs, and that we are doing a voluntary service . . . we have been activated and we are there to respond to these needs and in this way we can avoid conflicts. . . . It is not possible to deny that also in the last few emergencies there were conflicts because there is a voluntary service that is not ad hoc. . . . We need a return to the "popular" voluntary service that puts the ethic of the Civil Protection Voluntary Service in first place . . . and there has been no answer to this question" (male CPVS expert).

As always in this field, the opposite side of the question focused on positive behavior and relationships:

> It has been really good, although some situations, above all in Abruzzo, the ethnical difference of population and the approach was different, but I have not seen big difficulties for volunteers, I have seen critical situations . . . the relationship with the population was good, very friendly and the best one. [critical situations] The first one was adapted to different typologies of the population, but without a distinction it is a cultural question, we have experienced a cultural question, so we must be oriented in our approach and not offend someone with our normal attitude, I think the religion or the customs for the food and many other things" (male 1, province of Milan).

Other positive aspects were expressed: ". . .very good relationships, [the volunteers] became datum points. . . they are the facilitators, they listen to you, because they also do these things, they are not only operative, but they also have a heart and soul . . . in those situations she/he is regarded as a hero, . . . as important, and this charged up the volunteers (female 2, Lombardia region).

Listening to the population affected by a disaster is one of the fundamental actions required by the civil protection volunteers. Communication, the other side of listening, is a core issue that should be underlined as a social process in times of emergency and after the crisis: ". . .we have a duty to identify a group of people that is tasked with speaking with people, because sometimes there is the risk that all people discuss things with others and you must be careful because a sentence can be interpreted and said in one way or many others. . . . We are organizing this course because it is fundamental because the citizens who identify you as a helper must have your support, and so the responses are fundamental" (male, municipality of Milan).

Other reflections focused on the reaction of the population after the disaster: "Note that, in the last emergency, when you arrived there is the initial need, that is an approach by the volunteers and the earthquake victims because the latter are defenseless, they take all you can give them and [are] grateful for everything. And there are those who are in a difficult and shocking situation and so she/he can give time, things for a long period of time, and these are extraordinary situations and there are dynamics which are not always the same" (male, province of Brescia).

These dynamics can be analyzed according to the circle of offering and giving support and help by the Civil Protection Voluntary Service: "Yes, it is not necessarily a situation of giving and offering and getting something back; you can only give, and the people are happy and they have understood this action" (female 2, Lombardia region).

Human interactions and social relationships seem to be the core issue of the Civil Protection Voluntary Service:

> . . .this is the effect of the population on the volunteers, because when the population classifies civil protection as in first place, civil protection is all colored uniforms, yellow and blue, red, orange, green, which they see in action, but the splashes of color, it is enormous and always present, it is closer to the population, it collaborates with the population, they are numerous and present at the camps, they work a lot, and it is clear that interaction is required with these people because it is important not to forget that these people have lost everything. You should understand this mindset and understand how you can interact with them . . . because after a while we must go back home. . ." (male CPVS expert).

Referring to the Molise earthquake, the experience was positive: ". . .in Molise, where there was a small civil protection voluntary service, which drove the population to see that civil protection and its services were necessary activities and a culture of voluntary service and structure of voluntary service was created, and so this was useful as a voluntary service experience" (male CPVS expert).

Complexity and ambivalence are the main characteristics of this peculiar field of voluntary service. After a disaster, the population lives in shocking conditions, and they need someone who gives them the possibility of understanding what has happened and the ability to cope with the event. This is essentially based on the meaning-making and sense-making processes with respect to the beliefs that belong to the local population.

6.10 The Civil Protection Voluntary Service as a Resource

The final part of this analysis focuses on the type of resource represented by the Civil Protection Voluntary Service and the change in the relationship between all the people involved in a disaster. It is not possible to allude to the Civil Protection Voluntary Service without thinking of it as a multidimensional resource. In fact, it can be understood as an operative, technical resource, but it seems that in the past few years a lot of attention has been focused on the human and social resources of the Civil Protection Voluntary Service, according to the relationship that volunteers hold with the population, their colleagues, and leaders.

Furthermore, it is good to remember that voluntary service is the basis of the Civil Protection Department, and it is this element that strongly distinguishes the civil protection and civil defense systems: "Yes, now if something happens and there aren't any volunteers. . ." (female 1, Lombardia region); ". . .It is an indispensable presence. . . . Some years ago there weren't any volunteers except for the military and when something happened there were the military forces . . . the volunteers are indispensable. If they didn't exist, we would need other solutions or we could use the military again because there were no other solutions . . . they are all operative functions" (male, Lombardia region).

The necessity of the Civil Protection Voluntary Service was also highlighted by the male expert from the province of Milan: "In some sectors without voluntary service we would definitely close, because they are operative support and no other institutions could integrate their activities." Another expert noted that, "it is a fundamental resource, all civil protection institutions, national as well as local ones. Without the Civil Protection Voluntary Service, [they] could not have done what they did in Abruzzo and during other emergencies, because of the resource of the volunteers service; in Italy there are 1,200,000. They are people who do things and bring others with them to act and do everything that is necessary to respond to an emergency; 3,000 firemen do many things because they have training every day; instead the problem of the voluntary service is that they do not have training every day" (male, municipality of Milan).

The problem of training and the necessity of this activity to be in a better position to respond in cases of crisis and emergency is also emphasized by the diverse participation of civil protection volunteers. "It is an enormous resource . . . it is a structure that is now becoming very important, even if, unfortunately, I must say bitterly, that the State uses volunteers rather employs them" (male CPVS expert). The aspect of training demonstrates a reflection about the Civil Protection Voluntary Service in general:

> I think that the voluntary service has always existed . . . in my opinion the educational aspect is fundamental, it is an important resource that should be managed by important people, but the problem is that they are in need, because we need people who would be able to manage the voluntary service from a human point of view as an authentic resource. . . . I think we should return to a human voluntary service where people are respected and the volunteer is a person who should have more respect within the social field. . . . Today there is specialization, we are specialized in everything." (Female president of association)
>
> Nevertheless, the Italian Civil Protection Voluntary Service is at the core of civil protection activity in Italy. Italy is proud of its voluntary service. I mean, I remember a meeting with Japanese experts, when they had the destructive earthquake, the Kobe earthquake, and they are arrived for a visit to Italy and our organization of voluntary service and the fact, for example, that we are the ones that build the camp for first aid first. They asked us, "How much did the people pay to rent the tent per day?" This means that it is completely another culture. . . . It is the culture of voluntary service, a culture of voluntary service, I think, within which I deeply believe and it is bragged about by our international missions." (Male, Lombardia region)

What is important to remember is that, because of the actual civil protection system, it is true that the Civil Protection Voluntary Service is a fundamental resource, even if there has recently been a technical and operative vision of the unique activities done by civil protection volunteers. Instead, as some interviews have underlined, there are also other tasks belonging to the civil protection volunteers, including listening and providing emotional support to the population and helping in the aftermath and during the reconstruction of symbolic, human, social, and civil ties, which have been severed with the occurrence of the disaster – especially those with institutions.

6.11 Change of Relationships Typical of the Civil Protection Voluntary Service

The last question asked during these interesting interviews aimed to understand better the world of civil protection voluntary work and focused on the changes, if any, that have occurred among relationships, which are the main feature of civil protection voluntary work. In general the analysis emphasizes a big change in the past few years and specifically in this sector: "There is real difference because we have seen many associations implement their activities at the local level; instead, others have failed. We come back to the motivations because we choose to become civil protection volunteers, but also within a group, the internal relationships within the group and the leadership. . . . This is indispensable because if we lose the association it means that there has been no attention paid to improvement. . . . I think this is not useful and causes a split between the associations and the population" (male CPVS expert).

It seems there is also a radical change in the culture of civil protection voluntary work: "I think that there has been a big change, but less regarding the aspect of generosity and human feeling, instead the behavior, the training of volunteers has completely changed . . . also the management of the team at an emotional level besides personnel and among the relationships between volunteers. . . . This has been the real improvement of voluntary service . . . the results have been excellent and in my opinion they have enhanced the responsibility of the single volunteer . . . so, in my opinion, there is this sort of enhancement and awareness which increases the desire to give" (male, Lombardia region).

Other changes refer to the structure of civil protection voluntary organizations: "Nowadays there is a different organization . . . perhaps there is more responsibility, more maturity because today this is asked more frequently and above all not regarding the intervention actions themselves, but when you decide to exclude some volunteers from the intervention" (male, province of Brescia). Another expert stated: "I have seen the coordination of the system and the volunteers' activities, . . .they have had a different approach to the event, more shared, many teams . . . there is more analysis about the problem and the possible solutions, more sharing in the voluntary work. . . . So the response you give in that specific moment is more concrete, fast and direct arriving with many people and [without planning] you lose time starting to think about what to do, understand what has happened, and so the approach and the method are surely changed" (male, municipality of Milan).

Another expert argues that the role of the state within the Civil Protection Voluntary Organization has changed: "Before there was more spontaneity and perhaps less organization and preparedness, but surely more humanity. . . . The State has become too involved and it has created a bureaucratic structure which is too big. . ., in my opinion it is better find a direction of balance, mediation between the origin of voluntary work . . . and what they want nowadays as a good, precise, and organized voluntary work that nevertheless is not efficacious" (female president of association).

Another change to organizational aspects that is interesting within this analysis was noted by one of the experts from the province of Milan: "Since 1997 and until 2009, 12 years, the world of voluntary work has completely changed. In 1997 the system was building itself . . . the approach is completely different, the number of organizations, the number of regions involved, the typology of events, the years during which they have happened, there isn't a way of comparing, they are completely and fundamentally diverse" (male 1, province of Milan).

Deep changes have been made in the contemporary evolution of the civil protection voluntary organization, and many others relating to a different view of the civil protection volunteer could be realized in the next few years.

6.12 Final Considerations

This chapter has clarified many interesting questions about the issue of voluntary work in the civil protection field, as well as the possibilities for connecting these findings to the proposal of professional resilience belonging to all helping professions. By means of a sort of self-reflection, I asked what civil protection volunteers think about. To do this it was necessary to collect interviews from the civil protection experts and analyze them.

These interviews had the advantage of systematizing the previous knowledge about this field. In particular, they gave the future structure and useful categories for the construction of the online questionnaire and the arguments to be explored by it. The important issues listed below were specifically identified according to the general research project and its aim.

- Some personal data to identify exactly who the civil protection volunteer is
- The important motivations in the choices of becoming a civil protection volunteer
- The type of voluntary organization within which the volunteer is involved
- Who the "leader" of the voluntary organization is and how the decision process is managed

- The relationship among civil protection volunteers
- The sharing of rules handed down by the organization
- The role of the Civil Protection Voluntary Service
- A specific part dedicated to the relationships formed during the three earthquakes in Italy that were used as fieldwork for this research
- The relationship with the population affected by the disaster
- The evolution of civil protection voluntary work
- Judgment about their own civil protection voluntary experience

Following this structure, the online questionnaire dedicated to Italian civil protection volunteers is analyzed in the next chapter.

Chapter 7
Italian Civil Protection Volunteers: "Professional" Resilience and the Importance of Training

This chapter presents an online questionnaire for civil protection volunteers: its creation according to the dimensions explained by the semistructured interviews with civil protection experts, the pretest phase, its dissemination at a national level, and statistical analysis of the data collected. The online questionnaire was elaborated in three sections: the figure of civil protection volunteers, their motivations to become civil protection volunteers, and their organizations. A second section asked about the experience and various social relationships experienced by civil protection volunteers during three earthquakes in Italy, which are the fieldworks of this applied research. The third and final section inquired about the consideration and evaluation of the experience of voluntary service as experienced by the civil protection volunteers as well as their training needs in terms of disaster planning and management.

At the end of this analysis, the necessity of rethinking the role of helping and support played by the civil protection volunteers and their ability to be recognized not only for their technical competencies but also as "resilient agents" will become clear in a context of disaster resilience from a sociological perspective.

7.1 Introduction

After interviewing the civil protection experts but before analyzing their content, an online questionnaire was created and uploaded online using the Itstime web site (www.itstime.it). Itstime is a project of the Department of Sociology at the Catholic University of Sacred Heart–Milan, and it is the acronym for Italian Team for Security, Terroristic Issues & Managing Emergencies.

The online questionnaire was constructed with the aims of exploring the figure of the civil protection volunteer and her/his relationships with colleagues, leaders, and populations affected by disaster and better understanding the social dynamics present within the context of three earthquakes in Italy: Umbria and Marche in 1997,

B. Lucini, *Disaster Resilience from a Sociological Perspective*, Humanitarian Solutions in the 21st Century, DOI 10.1007/978-3-319-04738-6_7,

Molise in 2002, and Abruzzo in 2009. Attention was paid to the evolution of these relationships and in terms of best practices and response to emergency and disaster in the field of the Italian civil protection system, which was introduced earlier. In fact, using this method, it is possible to analyze disaster management and strategies of crisis and emergency management over time.

Before uploading the questionnaire onto the website, it was necessary to conduct a pretest to identify possible misunderstandings and to improve the questionnaire itself. Two sets of pretests were conducted with nine people involved in different organizations of the Civil Protection Voluntary Service (the municipality of Milan, the Civil Protection Voluntary Association, and the municipality of Paullo). These participants gave interesting suggestions for how to improve the final version of the questionnaire. In particular, they explained the different forms of voluntary organization in the voluntary field of civil protection, the range of motivations to become civil protection volunteers, and a better explanation of the research topic, specifically disaster resilience. Nevertheless, in general, the questionnaire and its connection with its aim was positively evaluated.

After linguistic and grammatical revisions, the questionnaire was divided into the following sections: (1) Social and Personal Data; (2) The Civil Protection Voluntary Service; (3) Three Earthquake Experiences: Umbria and Marche in 1997, Molise in 2002, and Abruzzo in 2009; and (4) Conclusion. The questionnaire was uploaded and available starting April 29 and responses were downloaded July 20, 2011.

The questionnaire was immediately disseminated by email to all civil protection institutions at local (municipality), provincial, regional, and national levels and all civil protection voluntary organizations. The result was the completion of 236 questionnaires. The following presents the findings from their data.

7.2 Section 1: Social and Personal Data

7.2.1 Who Are Civil Protection Volunteers?

The first section of the questionnaire focused on social and personal data with the aim of understanding the personality of the civil protection volunteer. For this reason the questions concentrated on the age, sex, region of permanent address, and educational level of the responders.

According to 229 valid responses and 7 missing values,[1] birth year ranged from 1939 to 1991 (Table 7.1). The year of birth of civil protection volunteers has a mode value of 1958, which equates to an age of 53 years old. In part, these data confirm the evaluations of the experts and the fact that the civil protection volunteer is an older person who often joins in the Civil Protection Voluntary Service because he/she are retired. However, today, people who are 53 years old may not yet be retired;

[1] This will be explained in Chap. 10 as there were missing values in many responses.

Table 7.1 Year of birth of civil protection volunteers

Year of birth	No. of respondents	Percentage of respondents
1940, 1941, 1942, 1945, 1986, 1991	1	0.4
1939, 1943, 1953, 1973, 1989	2	0.8
1944, 1951, 1956, 1963, 1968, 1972, 1975, 1982, 1984, 1985, 1987, 1988	3	1.3
1948, 1949, 1950, 1959, 1976, 1978, 1981	4	1.7
1946, 1960, 1965, 1967, 1979	5	2.1
1947, 1952, 1954, 1964, 1977	6	2.5
1955, 1969, 1970, 1974	7	3.0
1957, 1962, 1966, 1983	8	3.4
1971	9	3.8
1961	11	4.7
1958	**14**	**5.9**
Subtotal	229	97.0
Missing values	7	3.0
Total	236	100

rather, because of a change of lifestyle, the a healthy condition, and social and cultural changes, these people are now able to volunteer.

The year 1990 was not present. I explain the year of 1958 as the mode because of the baby boom that took place in Italy from the end of World War II until the middle of the 1960s. The other important value is that 11 people were born in 1961, which correlates with the same sociocultural framework considered earlier. What is very important is the nine people born in 1971, which marked the beginning of a new political and institutional paradigm, with the presence of new reflections about the welfare state, and its practical application. Furthermore, this was also a period of many changes in terms of the civil protection system and its application within the context of crisis and disaster management.

7.2.1.1 Gender and Civil Protection Volunteers

Another key point in this analysis is represented by the gender of civil protection volunteers. There were 234 valid responses (2 were missing), which demonstrated the following data: 201 were men (85.2 %) and 33 were women (14.0 %). This is important information that needs to be given specific attention because it underlines many aspects of volunteers.

1. The participation of women in 2011 at an institutional and organizational level: these data should also be useful for future analyses concentrating on the different situations within the European Union and across other nations.
2. When considering the different ways of processing decisions, the issue of gender is extremely important within the civil protection voluntary organizations and has a critical role in crisis and disaster management.

3. Leadership and gender is one of the topics within the sociological discipline of disaster; concentrating on the social and cultural aspects and the influence of socialization according to gender pattern orientation (Weber and Peek 2012), it is possible to identify different models of leadership, even if this practice is not structured and simple to define.
4. Because of the different socialization patterns, it would be interesting to explore the potentially diverse models of sense- and meaning-making within the context of disaster.
5. The issue of gender seems to be important within the internal organization of the Civil Protection Voluntary Service, but it loses its specificity during the context of an emergency and the impact period; after the first impact it assumes its usual differentiation, albeit not in a strong way, for the population affected by a disaster.
6. It also is possible to argue about this difference in terms of men having more time available to dedicate to voluntary activity than women; women have more things to do for their families, such as taking care of children and the elderly.
7. Another point is that civil protection is usually associated with a technical world, as an expert noted earlier, so it is possible that women choose another, different kind of voluntary activity and context, such as taking care of children, the elderly, or other vulnerable people.

What is clear is that sociologists are not uniquely interested in the biological differences between women and men; instead they focus on the social and cultural construction of gender role orientation. In this field, many research has been done by Enarson (2010), even though it is better to consider the importance of cultural differences and the sociopolitical context to which we are referring.

7.2.1.2 Regions of Permanent Address

During the interviews with the experts, they gave the impression of the importance of outlining the place of origin of the civil protection volunteers, with the aim of better understanding the influence of geographical and cultural aspects of the volunteer's place of origin. Italy is divided into 20 regions, and the civil protection volunteers who responded to the questionnaire came from 10 of those regions (235 responses and 1 response missing data) (Table 7.2). It was interesting to focus attention on these data and their meaning.

In fact, the problem of participation in the online questionnaire was present before it was uploaded to the website or disseminated through email, but these findings are particular because the process of dissemination was elaborated with attention to the possible value of missing data. Instead, the main cause of these missing data and their regions should be attributed to inability of transferring the questionnaire from the institutional levels such as region, province, and municipality to the operational level of the voluntary associations.

Table 7.2 Regions of Italy as place of origin of civil protection volunteers

Region	No. of respondents	Percentage of respondents
Lombardia	**202**	**85.6**
Trentino	9	3.8
Lazio	9	3.8
Toscana	3	1.3
Molise	3	1.3
Veneto	2	0.8
Marche	2	0.8
Campania	2	0.8
Puglia	2	0.8
Abruzzo	1	0.4
Missing values	1	0.4
Total	236	100

Many other points were taken from the data and analyzed (an analytical presentation of this question can be found within Chap. 10):

- The Lombardia region represents the origin of 85.6 % of responses (the mode of this analysis); this result is understandable because of previous contact with some of their experts at the administrative and institutional levels.
- The regions that are not represented are important: Valle d'Aosta, Liguria, Piemonte, Friuli Venezia Giulia, Emilia Romagna, Basilicata, Umbria, Calabria, Sicilia, and Sardegna.
- In particular, Umbria is absent, and this region was struck by an important earthquake in 1997 –one that was chosen as part of this research; there could be multiple reasons for this, but the main one is probably the need to move on and not to remember the earthquake. The same consideration could be applied to the Abruzzo region, from which only one person originated.
- Large regions in the north and south of Italy are absent from this list; more important is the absence of Emilia Romagna, which is considered one of the regions of Italy that is more attentive to civil protection issues. On the other hand, Trentino, which is another region that gives much consideration to the field of civil protection, is present in this analysis (nine people).
- Nine people come from Lazio; this can be explained by the assumption that the centralization of the Department of Civil Protection and the municipality of Rome are very focused on this issue, which probably is the reason for their high participation in this kind of activity.

It was interesting to focus on the gender of people who answered the questionnaire and their region of permanent address (Table 7.3). The distribution of gender as it relates to the region of permanent address showed that females make up only 13.3 % of volunteers in the Lombardia region, and only 0.4 % of females come from the Toscana and Marche regions. No women, for example, came from the south of

Table 7.3 Gender and region

Region	Gender (%)		Total (%)
	Male	Female	
Lombardia	72.5	**13.3**	85.8
Trentino	3.9	0.0	3.9
Lazio	3.9	0.0	3.9
Toscana	0.9	**0.4**	1.3
Molise	1.3	0.0	1.3
Veneto	0.9	0.0	0.9
Marche	0.4	**0.4**	0.9
Campania	0.9	0.0	0.9
Puglia	0.9	0.0	0.9
Abruzzo	**0.4**	0.0	0.4
Total	85.8	14.2	100.0

Table 7.4 Cross-tabulation of regions and final judgement of the personal experience of the Civil Protection Voluntary Service

Region	Final judgement about the personal experience of the Civil Protection Voluntary Service (%)			Total (%)
	Very positive	Positive	Negative	
Lombardia	**60.2**	26.1	0.5	86.7
Trentino	1.9	0.5	0.0	2.4
Lazio	4.3	0.0	0.0	4.3
Toscana	1.4	0.0	0.0	1.4
Molise	0.9	0.5	0.0	1.4
Veneto	0.0	0.9	0.0	0.9
Marche	0.5	0.5	0.0	0.9
Campania	0.5	0.0	0.0	0.5
Puglia	0.5	0.5	0.0	0.9
Abruzzo	0.5	0.0	0.0	0.5
Total	70.6	28.9	0.5	100.0

Italy or from Lazio or Abruzzo. It is obvious, then, that men make up the majority, with 72.5 % from the Lombardia region and 3.9 % from Trentino and Lazio; the 0.4 % of men from the Abruzzo region is the lower value for this modality.

Another interesting cross-tabulation analysis can be elaborated by contrasting the region of permanent address with personal experiences of the Civil Protection Voluntary Service. This analysis achieved about 89.4 % valid responses; 10.6 % of responses were missing data. These data are presented as percentages in Table 7.4.

Although the frequencies are low and, above all, the distribution is not equal, there is a large concentration of volunteers in the Lombardia region. It is possible to argue that, in general, the responses were very positive or positive and were negative only among 0.5 % from the Lombardia region.

Table 7.5 Educational level and civil protection volunteers

Educational level	No. of respondents	Percentage of respondents
Elementary school	4	1.7
Intermediate school	54	22.9
High school (technical or other)	**143**	**60.6**
Bachelor or master	34	14.4
Missing values	1	0.4
Total	236	100

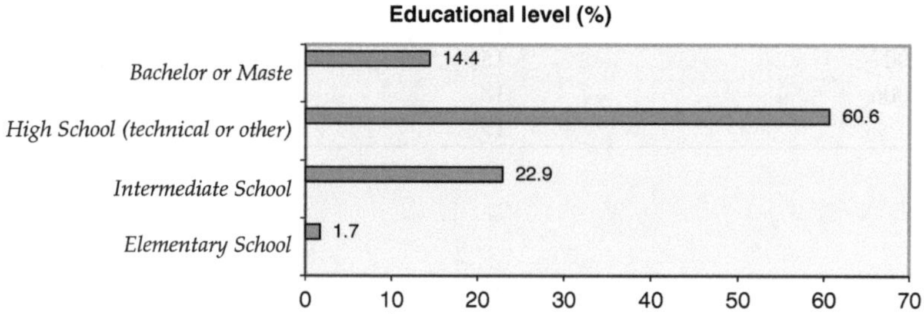

Fig. 7.1 Educational level and civil protection volunteers

These data could be interesting for future research projects, focusing attention on the territorial differences among all regions of Italy correlated with the diverse models of organization of the Civil Protection Voluntary Service. This could have interesting implications for adequate training experiences and operative and methodological reflection about improving useful models for civil protection organizations and their resilience.

7.2.1.3 Educational Levels

The educational level assumes an interesting aspect in this field, especially correlated with the hypothesis of motivations for becoming a civil protection volunteer, the distribution throughout the regions of Italy, as well as gender. The first analysis of this issue had various findings (Table 7.5). The mode value is represented by "high school," and this is a point of reflection about the possibility that educational level influences motivations to become civil protection volunteers. In addition, 22.9 % of respondents chose "intermediate school," and 14.4 % completed bachelors or masters level education. These data are presented graphically in Fig. 7.1. These data also are useful for future planning practices, proposing adequate training and courses, and improving the level (technical as well as relational) of both current and future volunteers.

Table 7.6 Year starting civil protection voluntary service

Year	No. of respondents	Percentage of respondents
1965, 1970, 1972, 1975, 1978, 1983, 1984, 1986, 1987, 1991	1	0.4
1968, 1976, 1979, 1989	2	0.8
1993	3	1.3
1980, 1985, 1988, 1990, 1994, 1996	4	1.7
2003	5	2.1
1992, 1997, 2001	7	3.0
2009	8	3.4
1995, 1998, 2010	9	3.8
2002, 2004	12	5.1
2000	13	5.5
1999, 2007	15	6.4
2005, 2006	18	7.6
2008	**19**	**8.1**

7.2.1.4 The Year During Which Volunteers Started Their Activity

The general institutional and political context within which the voluntary service takes place in Italy was described previously, and the fundamental questions, such as the recognition of the third sector, the laws that allow this process, and the deep influence of an Italian cultural background, were illustrated. For these reasons, information about when civil protection volunteers decided to volunteer is important as a general overview of this argument (Table 7.6).

Contrary to the historical and institutional process of the third sector and voluntary work in Italy, after a period of reflection about new models of the Welfare State, the Civil Protection Voluntary Service seems to be less developed in 1991 than, for example, other sectors of voluntary service. What is important to note is the concentration of participation since 1999 and, in particular, the years 2005 and 2006 (the mode value was the year 2008). This can probably be explained by relating it with other factors, such as increasing attention on civil protection issues in that year; the fact that it was almost 10 years after a specific law for the Civil Protection Voluntary Service, and, probably, the communication and announcement activities have affected the citizens.

7.2.1.5 Motivations for Becoming a Civil Protection Volunteer

According to the theoretical framework about volunteers and prosocial attitudes and the different motivations that have an important role in choosing to become volunteer, a list of possible motivations for becoming civil protection volunteers was elaborated.

Table 7.7 Motivations to become civil protection volunteers

Motivations	No. of respondents	Percentage of respondents
Offer help	**174**	**17.8**
Sense of civic responsibility	**159**	**16.2**
Possibility to enhance yourself	**114**	**11.6**
Donate something of yourself	86	8.8
Be a point of reference to whoever is in difficulty	82	8.4
Willing to live in a group environment	71	7.2
Generous	63	6.4
Have free time available	53	5.4
Listen to people during a moment of need	50	5.1
Possibility to enhance your professionalism	45	4.6
Grew up in a family where voluntary service was considered an important activity	45	4.6
Curious	16	1.6
Personal expectations	16	1.6
To adhere to religious values	6	0.6

The "other" choice allowed respondents to provide an open-ended response and add some personal thoughts. The list considered the following:

- Offer help
- Listen to people during a moment of need
- Available free time
- Willing to live in a group environment
- Generous
- Sense of civic responsibility
- Donate something of yourself
- Possibility to enhance yourself
- Possibility to enhance your professionalism
- Be a point of reference to whoever is in difficulty
- Grew up in a family where voluntary service was considered an important activity
- Curious
- Personal expectations
- Adhere to religious values

There were 232 responses and 4 missing values. These responses were analyzed using the multiple response procedures of the SPSS program. It was not possible to calculate the total value because the respondents could chose more than one item. Table 7.7 presents these findings. This analysis highlights that the main motivation to become a civil protection volunteer is to offer help (17.8 %), which confirms the social representation of altruism and the theoretical hypothesis of prosocial personality (Penner and Finkelstein 1998). At first glance, this is because a sense of responsibility has its role within the decisional process to become a volunteer (16.2 %).

Table 7.8 Educational level and motivation to become civil protection volunteer

	Level of education (%)			
Motivations	Elementary school	Intermediate school	High school (technical or other)	Bachelor or master
Offer help	1.7	25.3	58.6	14.4
Listen to people during a moment of need	0.0	38.8	57.1	4.1
Have free time available	5.7	22.6	64.2	7.5
Willing to live in a group environment	4.2	18.3	64.8	12.7
Generous	1.6	31.7	60.3	6.3
Sense of civic responsibility	2.3	23.9	59.1	14.5
To donate something of yourself	2.3	26.7	59.3	11.6
Possibility to enhance yourself	2.6	26.3	59.6	11.4
Possibility to enhance your professionalism	0.0	26.7	57.8	15.6
Be a point of reference to whoever is in difficulty	3.7	26.8	56.1	13.4
Grew up in a family where voluntary service was considered an important activity	0.0	13.3	60.0	26.7
Curious	0.0	31.3	37.5	31.3
Personal expectations	0.0	25.0	50.0	25.0
To adhere to religious values	0.0	16.7	33.3	50.0

It is also important to note the 11.2 % who chose civil protection voluntary service to enhance her/himself; this is perhaps understandable with reference to the circle of trust and altruism and the fact that altruistic behavior can be analyzed related to the theoretical view proposed by Moscovici (1994). Another interesting point is the dimension of giving (8.8 %) and being a point of reference for people in a moment of difficulty (8.4 %). The other suggestion that oriented the choice to become a volunteer is growing up in a family where voluntary service was considered an important activity and underlined by an expert is collocated to 4.6 %; therefore it seems to be not so decisive in this context. On the opposite side is the 0.6 % who volunteered to adhere to religious values. This data correlates perfectly with our contemporary societies and the processes of secularization and globalization.

Educational level is a variable that can influence the choice to become a civil protection volunteer. A cross-sectional analysis of educational level and the motivations for becoming a civil protection volunteer was performed (Table 7.8). A useful analysis was the single educational level where it crosses with motivations to become a volunteer.

For 5.7 % of respondents with an elementary school–level of education, the availability of free time was the main motivation, followed by 4.2 % who sought out the Civil Protection Voluntary Service to live in a group environment and 3.7 % who chose to be a point of reference to whoever is in difficulty.

People with an intermediate level of schooling chose to become volunteers to listen to people during a moment of need (38.8 %), because they want to be generous (31.7 %), and because they are curious (31.3 %).

Among people with a high school education (technical or other), motivations focused on a willingness to live in a group environment (64.8 %), availability of free time (64.2 %), generosity (60.0 %), and having grown up in a family where voluntary service was considered an important activity (60.0 %), which confirms the importance of family resilience from both a sociological perspective and as related to the voluntary activity.

The final group represents people with a bachelors or masters degree. They seem to have chosen the Civil Protection Voluntary Service to adhere to religious values (50.0 %), because they are curious (31.3 %), because they grew up in a family where voluntary service was considered an important activity (26.7 %), and for personal expectations (25.0 %). That 50 % of people with a bachelors or masters degree chose to become civil protection volunteers to adhere to religious values could mean that after receiving an educational degree there is also an advanced of level of abstraction in terms of motivation to become a civil protection volunteer.

In spite of this, it is not possible – as was assumed before this analysis – to divide the motivations to become civil protection volunteers into two macro categories: self-oriented and other-oriented practices. In fact, these data demonstrate that, in relation to educational level, the motivations among those with the same educational level are not homogenous; instead they are heterogeneous and involve both self- and other-oriented motivations.

Furthermore, an interesting correlation occurs between the variable of educational level and the variable of agreeing or not to the norms of the voluntary organization. This item was analyzed according to the correlation coefficient of Kendall. In this context the value is negative: –0.032, meaning that the relation between these two variables is opposite and that educational level does not influence the variable of agreeing or not to the norms of the voluntary organization.

7.3 Section 2: The Civil Protection Voluntary Service

7.3.1 Italian Civil Protection Voluntary Organization

In the previous section, the Italian civil protection system and the organization of civil protection voluntary work that has been present in Italy since the 1990s was presented in an organized and systematic way. In this context, the Civil Protection Voluntary Service is structured in different forms as associations and within local, provincial, and regional institutions. In the Civil Protection Service, there is no voluntary service; instead the work is based on experts' collaborations according to different sectors within which the civil protection activities are divided. This part of the online questionnaire aimed at exploring the organizational and relational aspects that are typical of these organizations.

Table 7.9 Type of civil protection voluntary organization

Type of voluntary organization	No. of respondents	Percentage of respondents
Voluntary association	**141**	**59.7**
Local group of voluntary service	72	30.5
Interlocal group of voluntary service	22	9.3
Subtotal	235	99.5
Missing values	1	0.5
Total	236	100.0

In particular, I analyzed the different types of voluntary organizations; the decisional processes and leaders within an organization; the relationships among volunteers during times of peace and times of emergency, which, according to the suggestions of experts, seem to be peculiar in this field; and the degree of sharing the norms about the organizations. All these issues seem to be important to understanding better the world of voluntary service and the social and relational dynamics that are typical in this context and to comprehending the possible proposals for intervention to enhance the resilience of volunteers and their voluntary organizations.

First I analyzed the different types of civil protection voluntary organizations because, according to the previous discussion about the general organization of the Italian civil protection system, I noted the importance that it assumed within the context of voluntary service. This question asked about three types of voluntary organizations in the field of civil protection: the voluntary association, the local group of voluntary service, and the interlocal groups of voluntary service (referring to many municipalities working together in the civil protection area). Of the respondents, 235 answered the question and only 1 had missing data (Table 7.9). The analysis demonstrated that 59.7 % are members of an association; this is interesting data, confronting the history of the civil protection system and the voluntary organization. In particular, this means that the Civil Protection Voluntary Service is an activity belonging to the third sector, with the typical and characteristic principles of this area, such as collaboration, altruism, solidarity, and civil responsibility.

An important piece of data is the 9.3 % of volunteers who work within an interlocal group of voluntary service; the interlocal group is a form of association that has formed during the past 10 years, although it has not had many successes because of the historical background and cultural features of the Italian municipality. This is also the reason for why 59.7 % of people join an association and 30.5 % choose a local group, meaning a civil protection group within the municipality. This can also be a reflection of the modality of information and dissemination that provides a horizontal model of dissemination through the associations instead of a top-down model that is typical of the institutional voluntary organization, as argued previously.

An interesting correlation was found between the type of civil protection organization and who makes decisions within the same organization. A positive Pearson correlation coefficient (0.179) was calculated. We need to consider that the correlation value is significant at the $P = 0.01$ level in a two-tailed analysis. For this reason, it could be assumed that the type and structure of civil protection organization positively influences the decisional process and leader within the same organization.

Table 7.10 Who makes the decisions within the civil protection voluntary organization

Who decides	No. of respondents	Percentage of respondents
The president of the voluntary association or the coordinator of the voluntary group with the volunteers	**106**	**44.9**
The president of the voluntary association or the coordinator of the voluntary group	68	28.8
Meeting of all volunteers or their delegation after group discussion	53	22.5
Volunteers	7	3.0
Subtotal	234	99.2
Missing values	2	0.8
Total	236	100.0

Furthermore, another interesting correlation was found between the type of civil protection organization and the maintenance of contact after the earthquakes. A positive Pearson correlation coefficient (0.183) was calculated. We need to consider that the correlation value is significant at the $P = 0.05$ level in a two-tailed analysis. For this reason, it could be assumed that the type of civil protection organization positively influences the maintenance of contact after the emergency and response phase.

7.3.1.1 The Decisional Process Within Civil Protection Organizations

The field of civil protection is characterized by the importance of the decisional process because volunteers are working in a peculiar context of crisis and emergency. This feature was assumed because of the information collected during the interviews with the experts and because of reflections about the context of intervention during a natural disaster. The circle of disaster includes a time pressure in almost all its phases, but not during mitigation and prevention activities, which are typical activities during a time of peace.

When asking respondents who makes the decisions within the civil protection voluntary organization, it was important to explore this decisional process for all phases and not focus on only a specific period of voluntary service. Therefore, four different responses were proposed:

- The president of the voluntary association or the coordinator of the voluntary group
- The president of the voluntary association or the coordinator of the voluntary group along with the volunteers
- A meeting of all volunteers or their delegation after group discussion
- The volunteers

Of 236 respondents, 234 responses were received and 2 had missing data (Table 7.10). The table shows that the model of the civil protection voluntary organization is based on a top-down pattern mixed with collaborative aspects: 44.9 % of people said that the decisions are made by the president of the association or the coordinator of the voluntary groups with the volunteers, but 28.8 % noted a top-down model.

An important aspect is represented by the last two choices: 22.5 % of respondents chose "a meeting of all volunteers or their delegation after group discussion." Only 3 % of people chose the answer "volunteers," which means there is little opportunity for organizational intervention among the volunteers themselves within the field of civil protection activities.

This issue also is correlated with another important issue of leadership in disaster. According to the current literature (Murphy 2009), leadership during a disaster orients and influences the success or failure of the crisis and disaster management, with specific attention given to the preventive and planning phases. Leadership during a disaster can be linked with many other interesting sociological concepts such as gender, socialization, culture, social relationships, and organizational process.

Leadership during disaster can underline diverse aspects of the same management: it can be instrumental or expressive depending to the social features and individual personality of the leader. Sometimes leaders can be associated with an images of a hero or a good person, but in other situations they are a sort of guide or "commander." What is important to highlight is the exceptional importance assumed by all leaders during disasters at local, provincial, regional, and national levels. Their collaboration is a vital element for the implementation of best practices regarding crisis, disaster management, and disaster resilience.

7.3.1.2 Relationships with Civil Protection Voluntary Groups in Times of Peace and During Emergencies

I now focus on the relationships among volunteers in times of peace (mitigation and preventive phase) and during emergencies (impact and crisis response). This seems to be a crucial point highlighted by the civil protection experts, connecting it with the literature within the framework of social vulnerability. This last aspect could be enhanced through the assumption that a collaborative participation within their own voluntary organization could improve the resilience of the community in which the organization is itself present.

The literature, especially the American literature, has paid a lot of attention to this focus, and sociological reflection has developed different social behaviors in times of peace and in times of emergency. This is a crucial aspect that all managers and disaster and crisis leaders should have as a key point for planning and performing effective preventive actions. For this reason, two specific questions were asked and the following answers were proposed (respondents could chose more than one):

- Collaborative
- Trusting
- Reciprocal help
- Friendly
- Conflicting
- Competitive
- Rivalry

Table 7.11 Relationships among volunteers in times of peace and in times of emergency

	Times of peace		Times of emergency	
Kind of relationships	No.	Percentage	No.	Percentage
Collaborative	**204**	**31.7**	**206**	**29.6**
Trusting	130	20.2	173	24.8
Reciprocal help	118	18.3	175	**25.1**
Friendly	**155**	**24.1**	**123**	**17.6**
Conflicting	18	2.8	5	0.7
Competitive	12	1.9	11	1.6
Rivalry	7	1.1	4	0.6

Specifically, many levels of all common social behaviors were proposed, taking into account the suggestions given previously by the experts interviewed. For the analysis of the relationship among volunteers in times of peace and times of emergency, the order of time in Table 7.11 is correlated with the order of the answer options proposed in the online version of the questionnaire. According to the table, in general, the relationships among volunteers appear in positive terms in times of peace as well as during emergencies; in particular, 31.7 % in times of peace and 29.6 % during emergencies. Other interesting and important figures are the relationship of trust (20.2 % in times of peace and 24.8 % during emergencies) and reciprocal help (18.3 % in times of peace and 25.1 % during emergencies).

These are interesting data because they represent the typical trends described by the experts; these exist in much other research: during periods of emergency there is more closeness and it seems that all negative attitudes are overcome to finalize the intervention for the safety and safeguard of the people affected by a disaster. In fact, conflict, competition, and rivalry decrease during times of emergency compared to times of peace.

This also means that it is possible to think about new sorts of relational patterns and the presence of attitudes that can contribute to enhancing a possible reflection on "professional" resilience as applied to the Civil Protection Voluntary Service. It is important to take into consideration the data about friendly relationships, which decrease from 24.1 % in times of peace to 17.6 % in times of emergency.

Because of this analysis, it is possible to understand this trend in this context; collaboration, trust, and reciprocal help seem to be functional attitudes both in times of peace and in times of emergency, particularly when time pressure characterizes all interventions.

7.3.1.3 Degree of Sharing Norms Within the Voluntary Organizations

Another important aspect within the civil protection voluntary organizations that is deeply connected with the type of organization and the relationships among volunteers is the degree of agreement (or not) with the norms of the organizations themselves (Table 7.12). The data from these questionnaires confirm that, in spite of

Table 7.12 Agree or not with the norms of the voluntary organization

Agree or not to the norms of the voluntary organization	No. of respondents	Percentage of respondents
Strongly agree	**131**	**55.5**
Somewhat agree	92	39.0
Somewhat disagree	5	2.1
Strongly disagree	1	0.4
Subtotal	229	97.0
Missing values	7	3.0
Total	236	100.0

Table 7.13 Type of organization and level of adhesion to the common norms

	Level of adhesion to the common norms (%)				
Type of organization	Strongly agree	Somewhat agree	Somewhat disagree	Strongly disagree	Total (%)
Voluntary association	**36.4**	**22.8**	1.3	0.0	60.5
Local group of voluntary service	17.5	11.0	0.9	0.4	29.8
Interlocal group of voluntary service	3.5	6.1	0.0	0.0	9.6
Total	57.5	39.9	2.2	0.4	100.0

everything, agreement with organizational, operative, and management norms is relatively high at 55.5 %. Although it is more than half, it is not a relatively large number (a range from 70 % to 80 %). This may be explained using the data that considered the presence or absence of conflicting and competitive relationships among volunteers.

What it is important in this analysis is that 39.0 % somewhat agree with norms, which demonstrates the previous hypothesis about the different quality of relationships and the typical interactions that exist among different levels – institutional, organizational, management and operative – of the Civil Protection Voluntary Service. It seems obvious that, according to this structure, the volunteers somewhat agree with the general norms characteristic of their own voluntary organization.

An interesting analysis using cross-tabulation shows the influence of the type of civil protection organization on the adhesion to these common norms. The analysis was based on 228 completed questionnaires, 96.6 % of which included valid responses; 8 (3.4 %) had missing values. There were no neutral responses. The data are expressed as percentages (Table 7.13).

Analysis confirms that adherence to the common norms of a civil protection organization is high for the civil protection voluntary association: 36.4 % strongly agree and 22.8 % somewhat agree. The same trend is also typical of the local group of voluntary service, with 17.5 % who strongly agree and 11.0 % who somewhat agree.

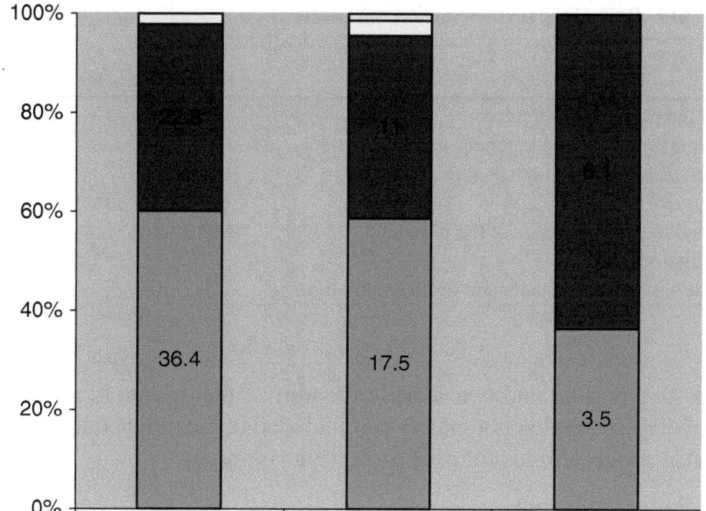

	Voluntary association	Local group of voluntary service	Internal local group of voluntary service
Strongly disagree	0	0.4	0
Somewhat disagree	1.3	0.9	0
Somewhat agree	22.8	11	6.1
Strongly agree	36.4	17.5	3.5

Fig. 7.2 Type of organization and level of adherence to common norms

The low level of agreement in general is specific to a new form of cooperation: the interlocal group of voluntary service. It is based on collaboration among different municipalities, sometimes involving 9 or 10, which does not seem to be a clear and functional model of the organization. Of respondents, 3.5 % strongly agree to the common norms and 6.1 % somewhat agree. In this case, the difficulties lie with the decentralized organization, which does not allow useful coordination of the civil protection activities. These data are shown graphically in Fig. 7.2.

7.3.1.4 Role of the Civil Protection Volunteer

After interviewing the civil protection experts, it was noted that particular attention is given to the different roles attributed to the civil protection volunteer. Specifically, it was observed that, in general, the typical role for a civil protection volunteer is within the operative and technical area; however, some experts underlined the role in the field of the population affected by a disaster, its management, and the emotional support from the impact phase to the response phase.

Table 7.14 Role of the civil protection volunteer

Roles	No. of respondents	Percentage of respondents
Assist the population affected	**204**	**24.5**
Disseminate preventive practices and behaviors	151	18.1
Provide technical and logistical management of relief aid	146	17.5
Respond to primary needs of the population	144	17.3
Train citizens	119	14.3
Provide emotional management of the population	69	8.3

For this reason, and considering the aim of this research, a question about the role of civil protection volunteers was included in the online questionnaire. Answers included different roles for civil protection volunteers:

- Training of citizens
- Assisting the population affected
- Responding to primary needs of population
- Disseminating preventive practices and behaviors
- Technical and logistical management of relief aid
- Emotional management of the population

It was possible to chose more than one response, and the final results are shown in Table 7.14. What was interesting in this analysis is the first result: 24.5 % considers the role of civil protection volunteers within the context of assistance to the population affected by a disaster. This confirms all the motivations that are the basis for deciding to become a civil protection volunteer, and this also is directly connected with the final aim that was previously illustrated within the Italian civil protection system.

An important value is the 18.1 % of people who consider the role of the civil protection volunteer as disseminating preventive practices and behaviors; this must be interpreted taking location into consideration: in Italy, the perception is quite different, and prevention planning at all levels (institutional, operative, management) is largely absent. This is, unfortunately, demonstrated by the three earthquakes considered in this research.

In Italy prevention is to be implemented regarding both natural disasters (and, for example, buildings, which often are not built in a regulated manner to safeguard the people living there) and industrial accidents or disasters caused by human action, for example, necessary training courses (evacuation, displacement) for the population living near chemical industries, which is almost absent in the majority of Italy, in spite of all the Seveso directives. It is possible to disseminate preventive practices and behaviors through preventive activities and simulations done with children and teachers in schools.

This is a plausible explanation because it is true that some courses are given to children in schools; however, in this context, these do not always occur and do not occur in a continuous manner or with a structured organization in all schools.

Table 7.15 Educational level and role of the civil protection volunteer

Role	Educational level (%) Elementary school	Intermediate school	High school (technical or other)	Bachelor and master
Assist the population affected	2.0	22.7	**60.1**	15.3
Disseminate preventive practices and behaviors	2.6	21.9	**59.6**	**15.9**
Provide technical and logistical management of relief aid	1.4	22.8	**62.1**	13.8
Respond to primary needs of the population	**2.8**	**25.0**	59.0	**13.2**
Train citizens	2.5	22.7	57.1	**17.6**
Provide emotional management of the population	**2.9**	**33.3**	46.4	**17.4**

Here the differences between North and South Italy are clearer, although the situation is not much better in North Italy.

Another curious result is that 8.3 % of people consider the role of the civil protection volunteer within the context of emotional management of the population; this is a small percentage but it highlights the future of the Civil Protection Voluntary Service. In fact, considering the civil protection volunteer only as an operative component of the Civil Protection Voluntary Service is a blind understanding because, as in many other studies in this field, the direction of this fundamental service seems to orient attention toward emotional and symbolic crisis and disaster management. In his masterpiece *The Human Side of Disaster*, Drabek (2010) underlines this position and suggests taking into account not only the technical and operative issues of the matter but also the human side of crisis and disaster that always exists.

Proceeding with the cross-analysis, we should try to understand if and how educational level influences the role attributed to the civil protection volunteer (Table 7.15). Some curious data emerged from this analysis. For example, among people who completed elementary school, the important roles attributed to the civil protection volunteer is to respond to the primary needs of the population (2.9 %) and the emotional management of the population (2.8 %). This is interesting in terms of training proposals for civil protection volunteers and understanding better their expectations and values as civil protection volunteers.

Quite curious as well are the results correlated with completing intermediate school. In fact, 33.3 % of people with this educational level think that the role of the civil protection volunteer should be the emotional management of the population; 25.0 % of them believe it is to respond to the primary needs of the population.

The real finding, which was anticipated, is the 62.1 % of people with a high school degree that think the first role of the civil protection volunteer is the technical and logistical management of relief aid. This is connected with what an interviewee said about this point: the civil protection system is essentially a technical and logistical world. However, 60.1 % of people think that the role of the civil protection volunteer is to assist the population affected by a disaster. Although it is not possible to generalize these findings at a national level, it is, however, possible to make a supposition according to the two paradigms presented by people with a high school degree: technical and logistical interpretation of the civil protection system and support for the population affected by a disaster.

The final educational level is represented by respondents with a bachelors or a masters degree: 17.6 % of people answered that the first role for the civil protection volunteer is the training of citizens. This is understandable through the assumption that people with a bachelors or masters degree give more attention to educational issues than other people. A similar number of people – 17.4 % – believe in the emotional management of the population, whereas 13.2 % of people think that the first role of the volunteer is to respond to the primary needs of the population. This is the lower value within this group and, sociologically speaking, it probably means that those with a higher degree of educational level believe that assistance to the population is possible through the use of other resources belonging to the people affected by a disaster and not only a technical and logistical intervention.

A final consideration should be based on the fact that the world of the Civil Protection Voluntary Service is heterogeneous and depends on many sociopersonal aspects such as age, educational level, and cultural framework of the membership. These can be important elements in the different training and educational needs within a civil protection context and as they relate to the different ways of responding to a crisis or disaster by an individual volunteers involved in various organizations of the Civil Protection Service.

7.3.1.5 The Citizen as a Civil Protection Volunteer

In the context of general voluntary service, one of the main topics is the participation of citizens in this prosocial activity and sharing solidarity with other people during a moment of difficulty in their lives. The issue of the citizen as a civil protection volunteer is a double-faceted topic. It can be understood through the paradigm of participation, civil responsibility, solidarity, subsidiarity; that is, following the sociological approach of Simmel (1995/1903), and the relational approach by Donati (2007a, b, c) during modern times. This relational paradigm has its own role in mutual relationships, which are the basis for a civil society and authentic human relationships. It can also be understood through a social and institutional paradigm regarding the improvement of self-help and protection, civil participation, and enhancing citizen's attitudes and capacities toward resilient activities and responses.

For this reason, the civil protection volunteers were asked whether they agreed with this sentence: "The first civil protection volunteer is the citizen herself/himself." It required a yes/no answer, and the results are discussed here (Table 7.16). Important data might cause us to rethink the Civil Protection Voluntary Service: 66.1 % of people strongly agree with the concept of a citizen as the first civil protection volunteer. It means a sort of cultural revolution within the Italian context because of the high degree of assistance that the population is used to.

This information could be useful in orienting future civil protection training activities and courses dedicated to citizens and in improving participation in the

Table 7.16 The citizen as a civil protection volunteer

Level of agreement or disagreement	No. of respondents	Percentage of respondents
Strongly agree	**156**	**66.1**
Somewhat agree	62	26.3
Somewhat disagree	5	2.1
Strongly disagree	5	2.1
Neutral	1	0.4
Subtotal	229	97.0
Missing values	7	3.0
Total	236	100.0

civil society, which in the past 20 years seemed to have decreased. These courses should be aimed at enhancing the activation of people in terms of individual and communitarian resilience for an appropriate response in cases of crisis or disaster. It could be a cultural passage from a welfare paradigm to a more active and participatory paradigm. Furthermore, this also means more collaboration between civil protection volunteers and citizens themselves in cases of emergency and disaster.

7.4 Section 3: Three Italian Earthquake Experiences: Umbria/Marche in 1997, Molise in 2002, and Abruzzo in 2009

Section 3 of the online questionnaire was dedicated to the three specific earthquakes in Italy, which were used as the fieldwork of this research project: Umbria and Marche in 1997, Molise in 2002, and Abruzzo in 2009. The section explored the experience of these earthquakes from the perspective of the civil protection volunteers who participated and were involved in the emergency and disaster management. In particular, it focused on the length of their intervention, their relationships with the affected population, the availability of resources by the affected population, the consideration of the population by the civil protection volunteers, and the maintenance of contacts with the population, including after the first intervention. These issues were chosen because I wanted to understand better what the civil protection volunteers thought about their missions during the emergency and disaster and how the population affected by the earthquakes considered their activities. A lot of interesting data was provided in terms of possible professional resilience, which has previously been identified in the context of helping professions.

7.4.1 Involvement During the Earthquakes

The first question asked of the civil protection volunteers was specifically oriented toward the experiences they had during the earthquakes and where and in which specific earthquakes they were involved. It should be remembered that it was possible for a volunteer to be involved in more than one earthquake.

Table 7.17 Involvement during the earthquakes

Involvement	No. of respondents	Percentage of respondents
Umbria and Marche in 1997	31	12.1
Molise in 2002	31	12.1
Abruzzo in 2009	**194**	**75.8**
Total	256	100.0

Table 7.18 Gender of people involved during the three earthquakes

Gender	Umbria/Marche in 1997	Molise in 2002	Abruzzo in 2009
Male	96.8	100.0	85.9
Female	3.2	0.0	14.1

The data show an interesting and deep reflection about the Civil Protection Voluntary Service (Table 7.17). Of the respondents, 75.8 % were involved during the last emergency – the Abruzzo earthquake in 2009. This is understandable according to some aspects; for example, the Civil Protection Voluntary Service has been consolidated and has become more structured during the past 20 years. Furthermore, these data are correlated with other two important pieces of information: the year of involvement (2008) and the region of involvement – information that was really useful. For this reason, the year of involvement and the region of permanent address were cross-referenced.

The analysis confirmed that most people who were ≥ 18 years of age and who became involved in the Civil Protection Voluntary Service in 2008 came from the Lombardia region; this was expected because the Lombardia region was represented by 194 people who answered the online questionnaire.

This data also correlated with the high presence of people from the Lombardia region in many civil protection permanent areas in Abruzzo and their role in management, coordination, and organization during the emergencies.

On the other hand, the low frequency of involvement and participation of people from other regions during the Umbria and Marche earthquake in 1997 and the Molise earthquake in 2002 could be explained by the process of development of the Civil Protection Voluntary Service. In particular, during the Umbria and Marche earthquake in 1997, the Civil Protection Voluntary Service was just being organized and becoming active; the Molise earthquake 5 years later was characterized by a high level of unknown procedures and disorganization in terms of emergency and crisis management, assistance given to the population, and coordination of interventions.

Although the gender gap is very high among respondents to this questionnaire, a cross-tabulation between gender and participation in the earthquakes was attempted. The data provide only an overview, and the meaning of the relationships between these two aspects should be enhanced by other research. The data showed the following trends based on valid responses of people involved in the management of the three earthquakes (Table 7.18).

Table 7.19 Duration of the mission

	Umbria and Marche in 1997		Molise in 2002		Abruzzo in 2009	
Time	No.	Percentage	No.	Percentage	No.	Percentage
1 Week	15	**6.4**	15	**6.4**	88	**37.3**
2 Weeks	9	3.8	11	4.7	53	22.5
Nearly 1 month	8	3.4	3	1.3	32	13.6
Up to 3 months	1	0.4	1	0.4	13	5.5
Up to 6 months	0	0	0	0	8	3.4
More than 6 months	0	0	0	0	0	0
Total	33	14.0	30	12.7	194	82.2

This table illustrates two kinds of interesting data. During the Molise earthquake in 2002, no women were present during disaster management in the role of civil protection volunteer, even though the Civil Protection Voluntary Service had existed for some years. Of those who participated in the Umbria and Marche earthquake in 1997, 3.2 % were women. There was an increasing trend with the Abruzzo earthquake in 2009: 14.1 % of volunteers were women. This last piece of data is quite interesting for consideration in future longitudinal research within this topic.

7.4.1.1 Length of the Mission

Another interesting question asked of volunteers was about the length of their mission during the earthquakes in which they were involved. This is particularly important not only for the organizational aspects and disaster management but also for relationships with colleagues and the population affected by a disaster. The data show that during all the earthquakes, the volunteers were involved for 1 or 2 weeks. In particular, 6.4 % were involved for 1 week in Umbria and Marche in 1997 and in Molise in 2002, whereas in Abruzzo in 2009, 37.3 % were involved for 1 week (Table 7.19).

The other important piece of data in this analysis is the 3.4 % of volunteers who remained within the permanent civil protection areas in Abruzzo for up to 6 months; this can be explained by changes in the mission and organization of disaster management.

In the Umbria/Marche and Molise earthquakes, the interventions were characterized by the displacement of people affected by the earthquakes into many different forms of dwelling, such as a tent city built by the Civil Protection Service, as well as containers used as homes and wooden houses. In Abruzzo, a decision by the president of the Council of Ministries, the institution that initially coordinated the Civil Protection Department, moved the population from tents directly to new permanent housing; for this reason people had to wait for 9 months while the new houses were built. The presence of the civil protection volunteers up to 6 months after the emergencies is understandable based on the knowledge of this institutional and organizational context.

Table 7.20 Relationships with the population affected by the earthquakes

	Umbria and Marche in 1997		Molise in 2002		Abruzzo in 2009	
Kind of relationship	No.	Percentage	No.	Percentage	No.	Percentage
Helpful	14	5.9	10	4.2	82	**34.7**
Reciprocal collaboration	15	**6.4**	16	**6.8**	73	30.9
Emotional closeness	4	1.7	5	2.1	27	11.4
Problematic	0	0	0	0	2	0.8
Distant	1	0.4	0	0	9	3.8
Conflicting	0	0	0	0	0	0
Total	34	14.4	31	13.1	193	81.8

7.4.1.2 Relationships with the Population Affected by the Earthquakes

The core issue of this research is represented by the social relationships between the civil protection volunteers and the populations affected by the earthquakes. The main focus of the analysis was to understand what kind of relationships were established. To achieve this objective, a list of possible types of social relationship was determined:

- Helpful
- Reciprocal collaboration
- Emotionally close
- Problematic
- Distant
- Conflicting

These typologies were determined according to the analysis of the interviews with the experts and the international literature regarding this topic. Respondents were able to choose more than one response (Table 7.20). The data demonstrated that, during the Umbria and Marche and Molise earthquakes, relationships were characterized by reciprocal collaboration, meaning that the professional aspects of voluntary service are a good basis for reflection about a possible professional resilience. Reciprocal collaboration has many aspects, such as enhancing and improving personal and communitarian resilience. As we will see through the interviews with ordinary people, their ability to be involved in the management of their own lives while living within a permanent camp created by the Civil Protection Service is important action to take into account for the future planning of civil protection management.

According to the changes in civil protection's management of the Abruzzo earthquake in 2009, the first kind of relationship was "helpful." This answer is fundamental to understanding the paradigm of welfare that emerges from the analysis. The presence of civil protection volunteers for 6 months and this "helpful" relationship is not a good basis for professional resilience because the role of professional resilience is to improve and enhance the resources already available or make them available to allow people to live in different conditions free from assistance and dependence.

Table 7.21 Gender and kind of relationship established with the population of the Umbria and Marche earthquake in 1997

	Kind of relationship with the population of the Umbria and Marche earthquake in 1997 (%)				
Gender	Helpful	Reciprocal collaboration	Emotional closeness	Distant	Total (%)
Male	38.2	**44.1**	11.8	2.9	97.1
Female	**2.9**	0.0	0.0	0.0	2.9
Total	41.2	44.1	11.8	2.9	100.0

Table 7.22 Gender and kind of relationship established with the population of the Molise earthquake in 2002

	Kind of relationship with the population of the Molise earthquake in 2002 (%)		
Gender	Helpful	Reciprocal collaboration	Emotional closeness
Male	32.3	**51.6**	16.1

Table 7.23 Gender and kind of relationship established with the population of the Abruzzo earthquake in 2009

	Kind of relationship with the population of the Abruzzo earthquake in 2009 (%)					
Gender	Helpful	Reciprocal collaboration	Emotional closeness	Problematic	Distant	Total (%)
Male	**37.2**	31.4	12.0	1.0	4.2	85.9
Female	5.2	**6.8**	1.6	0.0	0.5	14.1
Total	42.4	38.2	13.6	1.0	4.7	100.0

After analyzing the kind of relationships were established, I tried to relate these data with the gender variable to understand better the distribution of gender within the types of possible relationships with the population. Some interesting results emerged, as Tables 7.21, 7.22, and 7.23 illustrate. In particular, the differences in relationships during each earthquake and, through a longitudinal view, between the three earthquakes were reviewed.

The Umbria and Marche earthquake in 1997 was characterized by 44.1 % of men responding that they had reciprocal collaboration with the population affected by the earthquake, whereas from the female point of view, relationships were helpful with 2.9 % and zero for other kinds of relationship. During the Molise earthquake in 2002, among the people who answered the questionnaire only men were involved in the management of the earthquake. No women participated in the management of the event. In this context, 51.6 % of men established a reciprocal collaboration with the population affected by the earthquake.

These data and the interviews with the population make clear that, during the Molise earthquake, emergency and disaster management had a particular organization and logical structure because of the spatial context and landscape, the culture and

Table 7.24 Resources owned by the population

	Umbria and Marche in 1997		Molise in 2002		Abruzzo in 2009	
Type of resource	No.	Percentage	No.	Percentage	No.	Percentage
Yes, emotional	6	2.5	6	2.5	56	**23.7**
Yes, organizational	12	**5.1**	9	**3.8**	30	12.7
Yes, economic	1	0.4	0	0	1	0.4
Yes, social networks and friendships for helping	2	0.8	3	1.3	36	15.3
None	11	4.7	13	5.5	68	15.3
Total	32	13.6	31	13.1	191	80.9

traditional framework, the lack of an institutional collaborative pattern that made real management of the initial help and relief aid impossible, and, finally – but importantly – the emotional shock as a consequence of the death of 27 children in their school.

Relationships during the Abruzzo earthquake in 2009 were characterized as helpful for 37.2 % of men and as reciprocal collaboration for 6.8 % of women.

In general, support, help, and prosocial behaviors are associated with women. This is certainly true for the Umbria and Marche earthquake in 1997; data have shown a high proportion of women affected by the earthquake and who actively participated in the daily life of the organization during displacement. This helps explain the data related to the Abruzzo earthquake and the fact that 6.8 % of women indicated that their relationships were reciprocal collaboration. Enquiring about the kind of relationships among women volunteers and women affected by the earthquake to understand better their role in disaster management and their relationships with men would be an interesting research proposal.

7.4.1.3 Resources Belonging to the Population

Strictly connected with the kind of relationships between civil protection volunteers and the populations affected by an earthquake is a discussion about the presence or absence of resources typically owned by the victims of earthquakes. A question about this issue identified different types of resources owned by the population:

- Emotional resources
- Organizational resources
- Economic resources
- Social networks and friendships for helping

In addition to these, the response "no" was an answer choice in case there were no local resources available during any of the earthquakes.

The data provided an overview about the situation that civil protection interventions could face, depending on what they found once they arrived at the site of the earthquake (Table 7.24). The data showed a similarity between the earthquakes in Umbria and Marche in 1997 and Molise in 2002. In fact, 5.1 % of people answered that, in Umbria and Marche, the resources owed by population were organizational; this is understandable because during the Umbria and Marche earthquake the population was displaced many times into different types of dwellings, and it is possible that they possessed organizational resources in terms of moving to and reorganizing in the new accommodations. Only 3.8 % of people answered that the resources were organizational during the Molise earthquake, and this is understandable because of the moving that these people did, by their hosting relatives or friends, and the familiar resilience that was possible. During the Abruzzo earthquake, most resources (23.7 %) seemed to be emotional. In fact, much attention has been given to the strong personality of this population and of all the communities involved.

This analysis underlines the presence of few relational resources, such as social networks and friendships, through all three earthquakes. This is the core aspect of speaking about community and social resilience in Italy during natural disasters as well as those caused by human actions. In some cases this absence was presented and demonstrated by the interviews with ordinary people who were directly affected by the earthquakes.

7.4.1.4 Consideration of the Volunteers by the Population Affected by the Earthquakes

Following sociological tradition, the main topic studied from different perspectives was the social relationships within many various contexts. As we have seen, the social relationship between civil protection volunteers and the populations affected by disaster, is characterized by diverse dimensions. What it did explore was the consideration of the volunteers by the population affected by the earthquakes and the feelings of the volunteers regarding this aspect.

The volunteers were asked what they think about four "social images" of civil protection volunteers. The following were proposed as possible answers (volunteers could choose more than one response):

- A helper during a time of need
- A person who organizes and manages useful services and activities
- A friend
- A stranger

The data are shown in Table 7.25. Of the respondents, 42.7 % considered the civil protection volunteers as a helper during a time of need. It is important to underline that this consideration refers to a bounded and specific period of time – the time of need. This is interesting because previous analysis proposed the possibility of enhancing an at-risk population's knowledge of civil protection activities through the civil protection volunteers; instead, what seems to be more important are the activities of the civil protection volunteers only during the time of need. This consideration has practical and operative implications, for example, educational activities within schools or public meetings with the population potentially at risk. In addition, it seems that there is no real awareness about the opportunities offered

Table 7.25 Consideration of the volunteers by the population

Consideration	No. of respondents	Percentage of respondents
A helper during the time of need	172	**42.7**
A person who organizes and manages useful services and activities	112	**27.8**
A friend	102	25.3
A stranger	17	4.2

Table 7.26 Maintenance of contact with the population

Maintenance of contact	No. of respondents	Percentage of respondents
No	93	**39.4**
Yes, with systematic contact	40	**16.9**
Yes, for a short time after the emergency	35	14.8
Yes, with occasional contact	28	11.9

by the presence of civil protection volunteers in a territory potentially at risk for both natural risks as well as those caused by human actions.

The other image of the civil protection volunteer is "a person who organizes and manages useful services and activities"; 27.8 % of respondents chose this answer. A third major category (25.3 %) was the civil protection volunteers as friends. These data could also be analyzed according to the maintenance of contact with a population after the initial period of emergency.

7.4.1.5 Maintenance of Contact with the Population

Many people interviewed, both experts and nonexperts, mentioned maintaining contact with the population affected by a disaster after the impact and the initial period of emergency. According to the aim of this research, this aspect also was explored because it could become a useful and innovative sociological dimension to enhance the knowledge within the field of sociology of disaster and disaster resilience. For this reason, the civil protection volunteers were asked about whether they maintained contact with the population after the emergency. Four responses were proposed:

- No
- Yes, with systematic contact
- Yes, for a short time after the emergency
- Yes, with occasional contact

The final results of this analysis were quite different from what ordinary people said during their life stories (Table 7.26).

Table 7.27 Gender and maintenance of contact

Gender	Maintenance of contact (%) Yes, for a short time after the emergency	Yes, with systematic contact	Yes, with occasional contact	No	Total (%)
Male	13.9	**20.1**	12.4	**39.7**	86.1
Female	**3.6**	0.5	2.1	**7.7**	13.9
Total	17.5	20.6	14.4	47.4	100.0

The result was "no" for 39.4 % of people, and this is not comforting data if it is considered in the context of "professional" resilience in particular or disaster resilience in general. It probably was influenced by the short time during which the volunteers were present within the civil protection camps, which we have seen was 1 or 2 weeks at the most in the majority of cases. However, a good result in terms of hope and resilience is the 16.9 % of people who have systematic contact with people they met during the emergency. This is sociologically important data that should be adequately considered in terms of prevention and social resilience.

The gender variable also was considered in line with its potential influence on the maintenance of contact with a population after the emergency and after the earthquake's impact. Only 14.0 % of the total number of people who maintained contact were women (Table 7.27). Based on the gender of people who answered the questionnaire, it is not possible to make a correlated analysis between the two sexes; instead, it is possible to make some kind of comment regarding the trends among males and females.

The analysis showed that 39.7 % of men have not maintained any kind of contact with the population affected by the disasters and that 20.1 % of men have maintained systematic contact with the population. The same trend is present regarding women: 7.7 % of women have not maintained contact with the population and – different from men – 3.6 % maintained contact for a short time after the emergency. This does not seem to be good information within the discussion of social resilience and the key role assumed by civil protection volunteers during all possible phases of a disaster.

7.5 Section 4: Conclusion

7.5.1 Changes of Civil Protection Activities in the Personal Experience of the Civil Protection Volunteer

The three earthquakes in Italy chosen to explore the possibility of disaster resilience from a sociological perspective covered a span of 14 years. Crisis and disaster management practices and activities changed a great deal in that time, in line with the changes in the Civil Protection Service both at an organizational level and a legislative one.

Table 7.28 Changes of civil protection activities in the personal experience of the civil protection volunteer to today

Level of agreement or disagreement	Spontaneity	Increase in professionalism	More structured organization to respond to the emergency	Changes in type of help (both technical and listening)	More agreement with common rules during emergency response
Strongly disagree	**58.9**	5.1	2.5	12.3	13.1
Somewhat disagree	0.0	0.0	0.0	0.0	0.0
Somewhat agree	13.1	**39.0**	**44.9**	**40.7**	**44.9**
Strongly agree	7.6	**43.2**	39.0	28.8	24.2
Neutral	4.7	0.4	0.8	4.7	3.8

It was interesting to explore these changes, starting with the civil protection volunteers and what they thought about five dimensions that are particularly important with regard to changes in the civil protection system, including:

- Loss of spontaneity and rush of emotional enthusiasm as responses to an emergency
- Increasing professionalism and training for volunteers who are involved in emergency management
- A more structured organization of emergency response
- Changes in the help given: not only technical and operative but also listening to and supporting the population affected by disaster
- More agreement with common rules during emergency response

These modalities of response were constituted by the level of agreement or disagreement with these single items. The results are presented in Table 7.28, which presents only percentages to make the data easier to read.

For the first two items about the loss of spontaneity and rush of emotional enthusiasm, 58.9 % strongly disagreed that these changes had occurred. This means that we have many sociological opportunities to sustain professional resilience as it relates to civil protection volunteers.

On the other hand, the increase in professionalism – an important dimension in some models of training and in educational experiences of civil protection volunteers – 43.2 % strongly agreed that this change had occurred. This is encouraging, as is the other dimension regarding a more structured organization during emergency response (44.9 % of respondents somewhat agree).

Another fundamental dimension for sustaining the possibility of a sort of "professional" resilience among civil protection volunteers is the change in the kind of help offered to a population affected by a disaster, from not only technical and operative – which, remember, is a civil defense paradigm – to one more focused on listening to and supporting victims. Of the interviewees, 40.7 % answered that they "somewhat agree"; this "uncertain" response can be explained by the fact that, as an expert noted in an interview, the technical and operative paradigm still has a strong role, influencing and orienting the best practices for emergency and disaster management.

The idea of the importance and functionality of the interventions by civil protection volunteers is a basilar question, and it often originates discussions and conflicts between civil protection authorities and leaders and civil defense or fire department authorities and leaders.

For the last item – more agreement with common rules during emergency response – 44.9 % of respondents somewhat agree and 24.2 % strongly agree. This is a fundamental point within all different practices of crisis and disaster management. If the people involved, such as the civil protection volunteers, do not agree with the general norms that institutions and associations have established, it is probable that some conflicts or discussions arise; what it is worse, these occur not during the mitigation or preventive phases but during the emergency itself, when all resources should be oriented to the crisis response. At the same time, it is normal to disagree with some rules created by others, but what is important is that the general norms and principles must be respected to enable the right function and coordination in times of need.

7.5.1.1 Training Experience

Within the field of civil protection voluntary service, training and educational experience are necessary to enhance practices related to crisis and disaster management. Therefore, volunteers were asked whether they consider training experience important to helping their relationships with populations affected by disasters. "Yes" and "no" were the only two answer options. A total of 212 respondents (89.8 %) answered the questions; data were missing for 24 (10.2 %); 82.5 % answered yes and 4.7% answered no. The large percentage answering yes is a useful indicator for all people involved in the process of proposing training for civil protection volunteers.

Because of the many fields for which it is possible develop training experiences, it could be interesting to explore more deeply which kind of training volunteers expect, for example, simulation games, group discussions, meetings with authorities, or courses about social and psychological disciplines important during the initial impact phase and the emergency. This would more fully respond to the primary needs of the populations affected by a disaster in various contexts – not only technical or operative but also relational and supportive.

One example of this activity is the Civil Protection High School in the Lombardia region, which, since 2008, has been run in a structural and organized way, providing various courses for civil protection volunteers and civil protection managers. Other examples include similar schools in the Trentino-Alto Adige and Emilia Romagna regions; the former is linked more to a technical and operative model because of the influence of a historical German tradition on disaster management. Although there are some undeniable differences due to aspects such as culture, tradition, legislation, administration, and institutions, training experiences for civil protection volunteers is a core issue that should studied adequately.

Table 7.29 Region and training

	Training (%)		
Region	Yes	No	Total (%)
Lombardia	81.5	5.2	86.7
Trentino	2.4	0.0	2.4
Lazio	4.3	0.0	4.3
Toscana	1.4	0.0	1.4
Molise	1.4	0.0	1.4
Veneto	0.9	0.0	0.9
Marche	0.9	0.0	0.9
Campania	0.5	0.0	0.0
Puglia	0.9	0.0	0.9
Abruzzo	0.5	0.0	0.5
Total	94.8	5.2	100.0

Table 7.30 Judgement about personal experience

Judgement	No. of respondents	Percentage of respondents
Very positive	150	**63.6**
Positive	61	25.8
Negative	1	0.4
Very negative	0,0	0.0
Subtotal	212	89.8
Missing values	24	10.2
Total	236	100.0

To understand better the influence of the region of permanent address on the idea of the need for training experiences, data about this issue were cross-tabulated (Table 7.29). Interestingly, this data analysis showed that only the people coming from the Lombardia region (5.2 %) expressed no concern about the usefulness of specific training courses for civil protection volunteers as they relate to the management of relationships between volunteers and populations affected by a disaster.

The data also showed that training activities are considered important for technical and logistical issues and for legislative updating within the civil protection area or voluntary service field. The other values were low, but it is significant that not one person answered "no" when asked whether these training courses are useful and that the regions involved are where the earthquakes occurred: Molise and Abruzzo.

7.5.1.2 Judgement About Their Personal Experience

The final question asked about the civil protection voluntary experience specifically judged volunteers' personal experience. To do this, a scale was used, with answers ranging from very positive, positive, negative, and very negative.

A total of 212 respondents (89.8 %) answered the questions; 24 questionnaires (10.2 %) were missing data (Table 7.30).

In this context, 63.6 % of people judged their personal experience within the Civil Protection Voluntary Service as very positive. This is fundamental information when, for example, correlating personal motivations that tend to determine the period of activity of civil protection volunteers.

7.6 Final Considerations

This research was conducted in 2011, which was declared the international Year of Voluntary Service. Volunteerism is considered a fundamental service in our contemporary and complex society because of the number of people and institutions involved in the third sector and international changes in lifestyle and cultural frameworks. The third sector, as mentioned in the introduction to this chapter, has been a subject of civil society in Italy since the 1960s. It is impossible to ignore the basilar principles that represent the concept of civil society as a democracy through the free participation of all citizens, who have the time and are willing to be involved in solidarity, subsidiarity, civil responsibility, communitarianism, and support.

The Civil Protection Voluntary Service is one of the most important examples of voluntary service, in spite of its particular origin and features, and according to the experts I interviewed, it is necessary to enhance crisis and disaster management. Although it seems to have the same characteristics of voluntary service that occurs in other social areas, it is necessary to remember the particular work done during an emergency and the aftermath of a disaster. However, some fundamental voluntary actions can be distinguished as universal for all sectors of voluntary service. The more evident ones include altruism, empathy, prosocial attitudes, help, support, listening, and emotional closeness (Cohen 1992).

For all these reasons, I chose to disseminate this online questionnaire to all civil protection voluntary organizations after its problematic creation (see Chap. 10) and an organized pretest among nine civil protection volunteers chosen because of their membership in different voluntary organizations in the field of civil protection. However, the difficulties with disseminating this online questionnaire were due to the internal characteristics of the questionnaire itself and completing it as well as some limitations within the civil protection associations.

Taking into account my general aim for this research project, I sent the questionnaire to 236 volunteers. In fact, the possibility of interesting analyses that confirm some important theoretical assumptions made the proposal about "professional" resilience possible. The consequences of dissemination of and participation in the survey have, on one hand, show concentration in some specific social and personal data, such as the region of permanent address (the Lombardia region) and gender (represented mostly by men). On the other hand, the questionnaire is characterized by large differences in some information, such as the date of birth (a large range between 1939 and 1991), that made it impossible to do many cross-analyses without ignoring the large range of answers.

An important finding to underline is the change of the image of the civil protection volunteer as a hero: she/he cannot always be considered in this way because of her/his motivations that, sometimes, seem to be uncharacteristic of a prosocial personality (Penner et al. 1995) and result in certain actions, for example, maintaining contact with a population affected by a disaster. In particular, this refers to motivations that can be considered egoistic (improving professional competencies, social consensus, etc.) or self-oriented motivations, which differ from any prosocial motivations.

The identity of a civil protection volunteer is a multidimensional concept that is impossible to understand by choosing only one of the theoretical models presented in the introduction of this chapter. The volunteer's identity is represented by a mix of many aspects, such as:

- Personal expectations
- Recognition of their social role within the community (e.g., the issue of the uniform and its implications)
- Participation within their specific organization and their active participation in its daily life and its life during an emergency
- The specific competencies that should be required to become a civil protection volunteer (e.g., personality, organizational abilities)
- The consideration by institutions and populations: the main characteristic of voluntary service in all areas is that it is in a position between institutions, administrative agencies, and the populations in need
- Social support that they received from the population in need in particular and civil society in general
- Social support that they give in the form of help, emotional closeness, altruism, and prosocial behavior
- Willingness to be useful in their society (a sense of belonging to their territory and community)

All these elements are directly connected with the duration of voluntary activity and the creation of a stable identity role. In this context and in the civil protection sector, 8.1 % of people started their voluntary activity in 2008. This is important data because, according to the three-stage voluntary model of a volunteer's duration by Chacòn et al. (2006), they are in the period of stable construction of an identity role. According to this theoretical framework and its suggestions for understanding better the figure of the volunteer, the four previously created macro categories were considered:

- Prosocial personality
- Motivations
- Identity
- Culture and organizational context

These four categories were used to construct the first and second sections of the questionnaire, and the findings confirm the suppositions explained before starting the analysis. In our contemporary society everything is complex, as is the personal and social identity of civil protection volunteers. They are, in general, between 53 and 55 years old and have a high school level of education. This, in part, confirms the trend considering the civil protection world as a technical and logistical world. Also, most people started their voluntary activity in 2008; this is a useful indicator for future research within this field.

The second section again confirmed the fact that most civil protection volunteers belonged to a civil protection association. The failure of interlocal groups is probably due to the many logistical and personnel-related difficulties in coordination and organization.

Decisions seem to be made with a mixed model of collaboration between the president of the association and volunteers. This model leads to interesting considerations for the leadership within the Civil Protection Voluntary Service, and the best model distinguishes a time of peace from a time of emergency.

Positive relationships among volunteers of the same voluntary organization seem to decline during a time of peace as well as during emergency, as do volunteers' relationships with the population in need. Accordingly, the disaster situation as experienced by the population affected by the earthquakes was positively managed; this will be demonstrated later by the interviews with ordinary people. However, some of the population affected by the earthquakes thought of the civil protection volunteers as strangers. This would be a good issue for civil protection training because of its importance in a time of peace and during an emergency.

The third section of the questionnaire highlighted voluntary activity during the three earthquakes in Italy, and it is a sort of longitudinal analysis of the crisis and disaster management model of response and relief aid. Specific attention should be given to the Molise earthquake, which represents a peculiar model of disaster management, in particular during the reconstruction phase, but within this context it is not possible to generalize because each disaster is unique, with specific features and historical contingencies.

Attention must focus on the possibility of talking about "professional" resilience for civil protection volunteers. Taking into account its limitations – especially the lack of representation of many regions of Italy and the mostly male interviewees – this analysis showed that theoretical, methodological, and practical guidelines should be found.

Sociologically speaking, the civil protection volunteer remains a professional figure in the middle of the mission and professional paradigms. Primary and secondary socialization processes typically move people to become a civil protection volunteer. In this case, "professional" resilience is a personal and social attitude that is characterized ethically in the support of people living within difficult situations, with particular attention on their needs and the necessary response. Collaboration and responsibility are the major principles for this activity, but the well-being of volunteers means an intervention of quality with high implications.

Professional resilience is a social process that involves volunteers at different levels: other volunteers and the president of the association, the population affected by a disasters, and the institutions and administrative agencies, above all at national level, that coordinate disaster management. It means being a part of a relief and response circle of intervention, and it is characterized by prosocial attitudes and behaviors dedicated to the population affected by a disaster.

The analysis also has demonstrated the importance of civil protection volunteers in improving the small amount of resources available during to a populations during an emergency. For this reason the civil protection volunteer can be identified as a key figure of professional resilience, a sort of "resilient agent," according to different points of view: with colleagues in times of peace and with colleagues and the population affected during emergencies.

The methodological and practical implications are oriented to improve focus on the training experience of civil protection volunteers. The training should focus not only on a disaster's logistical and organizational aspects but also on the social process that is represented by a disaster. In this context, relational and social training courses to help volunteers better understand the possible relationships between volunteers and a population and their dynamics, with the aim of improving the "professional" resilience of the civil protection volunteers.

This analysis makes it possible to identify future challenges for this sociological paradigm. One challenges is changing the image of civil protection volunteers as useful and necessary only for a limited period of time, especially during the first impact and initial response phase of a disaster. Considering civil protection volunteers as useful and necessary people not only in time of emergency but also during all the other phases typical of a disaster process, such as mitigation and prevention, could be an improving and socially resilient process.

In fact, during a disaster, civil protection volunteers have knowledge of the territory and its features. This is one of the most basilar advantages in activating civil protection in a preventive context that dedicated to populations potentially at risk. Furthermore, prevention within this context could be considered as the main action in terms of decreasing social and environmental vulnerability, changing perceptions about this vulnerability, and at the same time increasing the "professional" and social resilience of both volunteers and the populations potentially at risk.

Chapter 8
Populations' Experience of Earthquakes and Possible Resilient Responses to Disasters

Chapter 8 presents and analyzes the 19 interviews collecting life stories from ordinary people who lived through the dramatic experiences of the Umbria, Molise, and Abruzzo earthquakes. This chapter explains the choice of life stories as an interesting method for social interviews because of their ethnographic and biographical assumptions.

The outline for life stories included three sections according to the different phases of disaster management: before the impact, during the emergency, the during the displacement and recovery phases. Various dimensions of the life stories were analyzed: life before the earthquakes, including social relationships, job, and family; the impact of and changes in life after the earthquake, the type of help received and offered, and the relationships between the population and the civil protection volunteers; and the displacement and recovery dimensions, which focused on the sense of community, place, and place attachment that determine disaster management and the future possibility of rebuilding. These life stories are presented as unique stories and multiple voices from each earthquake that was considered as part of this research's fieldwork.

The final aim of this chapter is to reflect on the disaster resilience process and how the social identities of earthquake victims are shaped.

8.1 Introduction

This chapter is based on the assumption that the populations affected by the earthquakes have interesting and important stories to tell to social researchers in terms of disaster resilience and disaster management. What the population lived through is a crucial experience in the life of the people involved, and it is a turning point, not only for them but also for the social community and its institutions.

Sure of this, I planned to interview people with the following characteristics who had lived through the earthquake experience: be an adult; have a lot of damage and/or

B. Lucini, *Disaster Resilience from a Sociological Perspective*, Humanitarian Solutions in the 21st Century, DOI 10.1007/978-3-319-04738-6_8,

destruction done to their house; and be displaced to a civil protection camp and then to another permanent housing solution for 2–3 months or more. These three are the only criteria used to select the interviewees; this method is related to the biographical and narrative approach in social science and, above all, it is linked to the methodological proposal by Bertaux (1998) and his ethnosociological perspective.

The term *ethno* means, as Bertaux describes, the existence of many different social worlds, each with their own subculture, within the same society. Applying a personal vision of and use for this approach, this perspective was extended to an ethnographic approach based on some particular aspects of ethnography, which are presented within this analysis as:

- Being with people (Madden 2010): "intimate contacts with participants raises issues of obligation, reciprocity, trust and the formation of friendships and again the process is one of a gradual building up of trust" (Madden 2010).
- The concepts of emic and etic within an ethnographic question and regarding sociological research using ethnographical tools.
- Interviewing people and the practices of negotiations and conversations: as Madden (2010) argues about negotiation: "it plays an integral part in securing funding, access to the field sites, explaining and setting parameters of research, committing to time frames and potential outcomes, and reaching agreement on the time and effort required from one's potential participations to acquit a project."
- Ethical questions about the right of the participants to include the research project.

The ethnographical approach is presented here according to these aspects, which are related to the identification of a researcher within the fieldwork, the access to the field, and the relationships established during the period of research – all of these considerations are argued in the Chap. 10.

During this analysis, attention focused on the images and descriptions of earthquake experiences collected from ordinary people and their stories about different phases after the impact; in particular, according to Bichi (2007a, b): "it is not founded on quantification of behaviours and attitudes of interest to the researcher, and for which s/he provides a definition which is the same for all the actors involved. Rather, it concerns the interviewee's social experience – relative to the phenomenon investigated – and therefore as the interviewee defines it."

In fact, it was interesting to try to understand their process of sense- and meaning-making and the ability to comprehend better if and how a sociological resilient process and its typical characteristics of prosocial attitudes and sharing of human and social capital (Dynes 2002) was present. I recall what was expressed by Quennet (1999): "the catastrophe is always a discussion after the fact that becomes part of the story, since it is not possible to comprehend a catastrophe in the moment in which it occurs."[1]

Unlike the social group discussed in Chap. 6 – the civil protection volunteers – with the population affected by the earthquakes it was not possible to gather information

[1] Quennet (1999): "La catastrofe è sempre un discorso a posteriori che si inserisce in un racconto, poiché non esiste catastrofe percepita come tale nel momento in cui irrompe."

using a questionnaire (online or in another form) because the difficulties of sampling, the time that had passed since the first earthquake in Umbria in 1997, and the possible mobility of the population itself after the earthquake.

The methodological approach of the biographical method within social science focuses attention on the stories narrated by people and their personal experiences, which are of social and sociological relevance. Life stories as a research tool was introduced by Bertaux in 1976 and then in other research in 1998 and 1999 they are also by bertaux. The main characteristic of this approach is the focus on a specific segment of experience: "when an interview is conducted, not on the basis of specific questions, but using prompts and probes to reveal the interviewee's world – in respect, that is, to his/her universe of meaning – it will be the account, as honest and complete as possible, given by a person to a researcher conducting the interview – of a segment of experience or an entire life course. It will be constituted by what that person chooses to tell, what s/he remembers and wants others to know (Bichi 2002). We will recognize the presence of these three elements in all three fieldworks: (1) what the person chooses to tell; (2) what she/he remembers; and (3) what she/he wants others to know.

According to this research and scientific proposal, this approach placed the interviews within the framework of nondirective typology with the following features, as described by Bichi (2007a, b): a low level of standardization; various but nevertheless low levels of directiveness; and a high degree of structuring in the outline. This method was chosen because the aim was to understand the personal and sociological meaning of an earthquake experience, not through the words of experts, public administrators, or other institutional people but through ordinary people and all the difficulties they lived through during the aftermath and now that the emergency has passed.

An interesting question about the single world stricken by the earthquake and the dynamics of responding in an adequate way to survive and try to live again as before the disaster. For this reason, it was assumed that all the human and emotional information collected through the use of this method could not possibly be collected in another manner.

All the people interviewed are Italians (this point will be discussed later). One consideration should be noted: these interviewees' language was rich in terms of images, feelings, emotions, etc., in comparison with the experts interviewed earlier. Another difference was that experts are sometimes "constricted" to answer in a way that represents the institutional and administrative organization within which they work. This is a fundamental distinction between these two social groups as a focus of this analysis, but the main difference is the direct and indirect experience of earthquake.

The method used for this analysis was influenced by the approach proposed by Bertaux (1976, 1999), in particular, for the importance attributed to three functions of a life story:

1. *Explorative function:* it is a moment during which the researcher explores the different conceptions and realities of the argument that she/he has chosen to study. The interview is not a complete life story; instead it seems more like a simple interview to understand better the fieldwork and research.
2. *Analytical function:* The analysis of the first interviews is interesting and can orient the next interviews and how to conduct them. During this phase, as Bertaux

(1999) argued, it is possible to comprehend better the inner workings and the typical dynamics of the object of study and research. Bertaux suggests that this phase is concluded when the interviews do not reveal other interesting dynamics and the researcher understands the general course of the argument in which she/he is interested.

3. *Expressive function:* Bertaux (1999) argues that the complete transcription of a life story is not necessary because the communication of the story itself also has to be considered.

The other very important characteristic of this approach is the value of listening. It is quite impossible to collect a life story without showing interest in the story told by the person in front of you. It is better not to undervalue the importance of listening within the context of a life story and its collection, but this and other methodological issues are discussed in Chap. 10.

8.2 Outline for the Life Story

The outline for the life story is characterized by (Bichi 2007a, b): "the interview outline does not have always a direct interrogative function: not always, that is to say, is the outline used as a written list of the questions to be asked – a list read by the interviewer (and/or by the interviewee) in a more or less standardized manner." In fact, the outline in the context of a life story is used as a guideline of arguments that the researcher should talk about with the interviewee, but not, as noted above, in a direct manner; instead it must facilitate the memory of the interviewee and encouraging her/him to talk about the questions with the researcher. This is not a semistructured interview with the aim of collecting useful information to orient a future research project; instead it is an interview in the form of a story because we are interested, as researchers and as people, in what others have to say to us. For this reason, the following outline was created, based on the first introduction to the life story.

> Would you tell me, please, your earthquake experience, starting with the description of your life and its organization (family, job, hobbies, friends) 1 year before the earthquake itself?

A description of their experience about the earthquake 1 year before the earthquake itself was chosen as a starting point because it seems to be a good point to try to understand the life changes that occurred before and after the earthquake experience. Furthermore, especially considering the Umbria earthquake in 1997, it was not adequate to return to facts older than 15 years. It has the typical form of a life story that is oriented to the story of a specific segment of life, as Bertaux (1999) suggests.

However, the outline was created considering the same basilar arguments explored through the interviews with the population and was divided according to the circle of disaster and its phases:

1. Time before the earthquake
    1.1. Family: previous experience of an earthquake
    1.2. Job
    1.3. Social relationships (social networks, community)
    1.4. Hobbies, interests
    1.5. Perception and memory about known places, spaces, house/home
    1.6. Existence of previous contacts with civil protection volunteers or knowledge of the Civil Protection System
2. The impact of the earthquake
    2.1. The first response to the emergency: immediate actions and behaviors
    2.2. The first help received: from whom, what it was, and its duration
    2.3. The first help offered: to whom, what it was, and its duration
    2.4. Perception and memory linked to the space and time of the critical event
    2.5. Past and present social relationships as resources for emergency response
3. The immediate period after impact and the response to the emergency
    3.1. The first contact with civil protection volunteers: how? when? where?
    3.2. The figure of the civil protection volunteer during the first phases of the emergency response: description and characteristics of the relationship established
    3.3. Past and present interpersonal and social relationships and their changes
4. After the impact
    4.1. New habitation within the civil protection area (mobility, organization, legitimacy, social and institutional recognition): established relationships with civil protection volunteers, space perception (institutional and not), typology and characteristics, new experienced identity
    4.2. Community perception and living together in the habitation prepared by civil protection: perception and experience of attitudes such as cohesion, collaboration, conflict, and social distance during the time together
    4.3. Old and new interpersonal and social relationships: changes and characteristics
    4.4. Image and role of civil protection volunteers during this phase
5. Reconstruction
    5.1. New location and habitation
    5.2. Resources used during reconstruction: typology, characteristics, and availability

5.3. Help provided and received: to/from whom, what it was, its duration (perception of help)
5.4. Image and role of civil protection volunteers during this phase

6. Reconstruction/Mitigation

6.1. New organization of life and its changes
6.2. Social relationships and their changes
6.3. Experience for the future: training

Attention is focused on some crucial issues found during previous interviews to understand better the social dynamics and the possible resilient paths that people used before, during, and after the earthquakes. In general, the arguments can be summarized as follows:

- Life before the earthquake and the importance of the presence or absence of social relationships as social capital and previous knowledge of the civil protection voluntary system and civil protection volunteers
- Help received and offered to better understand and define the role of civil protection volunteers as a resilient element of crisis and disaster management
- The definition of and feelings about civil protection volunteers
- Displacement and new forms of housing (tents, civil protection area, temporary housing such as containers and wooden houses)
- Change in spatial perception
- Life changes and the consequences after the earthquake
- Availability of resources and their typology
- Old and new personal and social relationships
- New location and the perception of the link with the past, also in terms of spatial organization and memory
- Future expectations and the best reconstruction practices
- Importance of training for the population potentially at risk

These are general categories that were talked about with the people interviewed. One of the other considerations is that in the first version of the outline of a life story, the space and place components were not considered as being as important within this exploration, but after three interviews these were understood as indeed being important. This argument is also important according to the spatial and historical memory that is attributed to the places where people live.

Finally, this part of the empirical research was based on the aim expressed by Kaniasty (2011, 2012) "we need to find ways to support people in disaster-affected communities so they can help one another and disaster doesn't just affect the physical environment but the very nature and structure of affected communities so rebuilding efforts need to involve rebuilding a sense of community and re-connecting people to each other as well as rebuilding the infrastructure."[2]

---

[2] http://www.psychology.org.au/Content.aspx?ID=3956.

8.3 Umbria Earthquake in 1997

The event of the Umbria-Marche earthquake in 1997 was described previously. In the following section, an analysis of the experience lived through by people and recounted by them in the Umbria region chosen for fieldwork is shown.

Seven people were interviewed the Umbria earthquake: 5 women (two were 40 years old and the others were 48, 46, and 41 years old) and 2 men (41 and 68 years old). All of them gave an interpretation of the earthquake, on one hand in terms of natural forces or entities and on the other according to some ancestral and traditional images. For example, the 68-year-old man noted that "the earthquake does not break the houses, but ruins man" and "with the earthquake is a concentration of problems."

As mentioned above, another vision is based on the natural entities involved with and sensations felt during the earthquake: "that night it was terrible. . ., there was a boom that seemed like the end of the world" (female, 48 years old); "I did not understand anything, booms, booms from everywhere" (female, 40 years old); and "it was not the earthquake, therefore, for me, it was someone in my house, . . . that shook the bed" (female, 41 years old). According to these brief descriptions of the earthquake, the feelings about this natural disaster concentrate on the physical sensations and the difficulties of interpreting and orienting adequate behaviors in the critical context.

The fear of an earthquake came some months before: "when I felt the first shakes I remembered and I did not sleep during the night" (female, 46 years old); "you already felt that it was an anomalous thing" (female, 46 years old).

Within these words there is all the sorrow, pain, and difficulty of understanding the situation and the impossibility of believing what happened. This is an important point for sociological resilience in terms of awareness of earthquake risk and the knowledge of appropriate behaviors in cases of an emergency or natural disaster. In fact, these simple words help to confirm the necessity of training for the populations that live in areas that are potentially at risk for both natural or industrial emergencies. They explain the need to orient specific training programs to create a common cognitive framework, within which it is possible to collocate a common experience of crises, emergencies, and disasters. It is also important to take into consideration the importance of the single world of meaning of the people who could be affected by earthquakes or disasters in general.

The difficulty of understanding the physical phenomena of an earthquake was expressed well: "before the frequent and strange shakes were the booms" (female, 40 years old). Ordinary people do not have adequate information about natural disasters, especially earthquakes, even if they live in a geographically seismic area. In spite of this, people asked for more communication and information: "if only they had said, 'If there are shakes do this,' because we did not know how to behave" (female, 46 years old).

This not only underlines the deep necessity of training and information for the population to allow all people at risk an active role during an emergency but also represents the urgent necessity to think about the vulnerability of institutions and a lack of communication systems; at a local level, these could be represented by the local group of civil protection volunteers within the structure of the municipality or in the form of an association of the third sector.

After the first phase of the impact and all the destruction, physical and symbolic, caused by the earthquake, the population is disoriented and does not have the behavioral skills to act immediately in a resilient way: "during those moments, you do not understand" (female, 40 years old); "I had not realized that it was the earthquake" (female, 41 years old); "you get nowhere" (female, 40 years old). Within this specific phase of a disaster, people are completely upset: "we were not able to speak to each other, everyone had trembling mouths" (female, 48 years old).

The feelings of disorientation and confusion also are high because "it was such a big tragedy" (female, 48 years old); there were "strange and uncontrollable reactions" (female, 48 years old); and it was "an impressive thing . . . I was alone with the children and so it was even more tragic" (female, 41 years old).

They continued: "we were all around and wandered like zombies" (female, 46 years old); "we lost everything" (female, 40 years old), and "everything was interrupted" (female, 48 years old). This feeling of interruption and loss also is presented according to spatial and temporal questions: "from one moment to another" (female, 48 years old); "it is terrible because you don't have the physical place of memories" (female, 48 years old) because "the place evokes personal feelings" (female, 48 years old).

It is clear from these statements that the importance of feelings related to places and belonging were the main characteristics of this earthquake and the population affected by it. It also represents a model of the sociological resilience process, based on strong communitarian identities of the people affected and their willingness to live in the same place as before the earthquakes. This could also be a cultural characteristic of Western societies; for example, after the Sichuan earthquake in 2008, the people and authorities decided to rebuild in an area different than the one stricken by the earthquake.

During these moments people are confused and in a state of denial: "because then there is the refusal to see things as they are" (female, 46 years old), and "a series of problems trigger off which are not simple to face" (female, 46 years old). For example, there is lack of information and people who could help in terms of meaning-making during this critical situation, and that lack remains: "I knew only that I could not come back home . . . therefore life stopped" (female, 46 years old).

Finally, there is no better way to conclude this section about earthquake experiences than using the following words: "because then you have fear, you think that at any moment it really will fall down, the earth will open and swallow you, because this is the effect of the earthquake, that is, every moment you think, 'everything will stop, I will not be there'; it is a sensation of impotence" (female, 46 years old).

8.3.1 The Period After the Emergency

A generally important consideration to explain in this context is the impossibility of reproducing the analysis of the interviews in the same way as the outline of the interview itself; in fact, the interviews do not follow the temporal division of the outline, but the same phases overlap, probably because of the difficulty in remembering this dramatic experience lived through 14 years ago.

According to the crisis and disaster model of management there are some characteristics of this earthquake to be considered. First, the Civil Protection Voluntary Service was not present as a stable organization and structure; during those years the Civil Protection Voluntary Service was just becoming a fundamental component within the Italian civil protection system. Second, disaster management and displacement were managed through different systems of temporary housing: tents within the civil protection area, caravans, containers (used as temporary housing), and wooden temporary houses. This is important to take into account because the system of displacement orients and constructs different ways of responding to the aftermath of the earthquake with respect to the population and for their places of living. The following quotes demonstrate this: "the people wanted to remain living here" (female, 48 years old); "the fact that the people did not move on" (female, 48 years old) is important because they are "attached to the homeland, to [their] roots" (female, 48 years old).

This aspect, linking to the importance of the place of birth and the homeland, in general, also is visible within the earthquake experience lived through by older people. "If you take an elderly person and you move her/him far away, it is like homicide" (male, 68 years old); in addition, "oddities by the elderly" (female, 40 years old) were noted.

The argument of the link between older people and the place of living is a sociological theme of enormous relevance, above all in the context of displacement after an emergency and safeguarding a healthy life for the elderly. This consideration has practical implications in terms of disaster management and the recognition of personal and individual vulnerability that specifically belongs to older people, which should be faced with the collaboration and participation of institutional agencies and the population in an attempt to find the best solution possible while considering the availability of various resources (individual, familiar, economical, communitarian).

8.3.2 *The Image of the Civil Protection Volunteer and the Population: Received and Offered Help*

The sociological resilient process during a natural disaster could be based on circular actions of supporting and helping among the population, the civil protection volunteers, and the institutional agencies that must respond to a crisis and emergency. The first analysis of these interviews and those for the Molise and Abruzzo earthquakes confirmed that resilience is an individual attitude supported and oriented by the community and society within which a person lives. For this reason, sociological resilience can be considered through the assumption of four different dimensions: personal and individual, familiar, communitarian, and social.

In particular, it seems that less of a role can be attributed to institutional and organizational resilience, which are basilar for better disaster management but seem not to be adequately developed within the Italian context; instead they seem to be removed from the whole circle of sociological resilience for natural disaster management.

As stated earlier, it was not possible to follow the timeline presented in the outline while interviewing because of a change within the perception and memory of the people affected by the earthquakes; the telling of their experience was characterized by often returning to another point in the story, not in linear way but through stopping and continuing. For this reason, the analysis and interpretation of the information collected follows only one big section in which it is possible find descriptions of the experience lived through after the emergency, the period during which civil protection volunteers were present, and the actions to rebuild and reconstruct. In this context, it is true that the researcher has the role of aide-mémoire, but it was not simply to try to make up a story with a perfect timeline; instead the memory follows the symbolic images of earthquake experiences, but it was possible to collect an interesting suggestion of how to comprehend sociological resilience in natural disasters.

The aftermath is a period of confusion and disorientation; many people reacted in ways that are misunderstood by others, and the interviewees underline the fact that there were "changed people" (female, 40 years old) and that "everyone reacts in their own way" (female, 40 years old). This period of time can vary in different ways that are due to the model chosen for crisis and emergency management, the community and the population stricken by the disaster, and the internal characteristics of the population itself. But there are also some universal features that lie more in the anthropological vision. In this context these are represented by the statement, "during the emergency there are those who become kinder and more good and those who become greedier" (female, 46 years old). Many people change during the aftermath and while living in temporary shelters, and this is a real fact that should be analyzed and considered by sociologists as well as social scientists.

In general, the ambivalence of behaviors are represented by two quite opposite positions: on one hand there are people who "try to do things not think about everything" (female 40 years old); on the other hand, ". . .some prefer to be waited on hand and foot" (female 41 years old). The concrete problem is finding a way to guarantee an acceptable level of "collaboration and patience from the people" (female, 48 years old) through the effort to "carry forward all the solutions to satisfy almost all the people" (male, 68 years old).

It is known that conflicts and difficult dynamics are present during all types of disasters and emergencies, but working within a collaborative as well as participative context is necessary for civil protection volunteers, the Civil Protection System, and institutional agencies. Sometimes, as we have unfortunately seen with the Abruzzo earthquake in 2009, these two important aspects – collaboration and participation from the population – are not well supported by institutional agencies. As a result, the phases after impact as a response to the emergency and reconstruction have a high percentage of conflicts that do not allow the process to focus on the real problems and needs revealed by the population affected. Sometimes the needs of the people affected by a disaster are not deeply considered. For example, "the thing that really exhausts you is the long waiting, the long times" (female, 46 years old).

Feelings of frustration and impotence are present in many people, and future training courses for both civil protection volunteers and institutional personnel should teach ways to manage them. This aspect is underlined "because, in my opinion, during the emergency you need technicians not politicians" (female, 46 years old). The issue is not only about the specific and professional role of technicians and politicians but the fact that, when such sensitive issues cross the path of politics, everyone assumes a position that does not function during the response to and reconstruction after the earthquake.

Within this context of destruction, sorrow, and desperation the civil protection volunteer supposedly plays a central role in the response to a disaster through a resilient experience. This is true regarding the Umbria earthquake, but the volunteers did not belong to the Civil Protection System; instead, they came from different associations of the third sector and voluntary service, such as Caritas: "with the coming of volunteers . . . from Caritas let us say it was a turning point of the situation, because if you are really alone you are unable to go on" (female, 46 years old). They were a turning point during this period and played the role of interconnection between the population, its needs, and the institutional system of emergency and disaster management.

It is necessary to remember that, during those years, the voluntary service in Italy began to be part of the development of the welfare state, but it was at the beginning of its service: "the discourse of civil protection and voluntary service was started immediately after" (female, 46 years old). For this reason, it can be argued that the sociological resilient process was not simply focused on received and offered help. Instead it is in large part based on personal and individual attitudes that were shared within the community of belonging, and the civil protection volunteers had the tasks and goal of facilitating and negotiating this process to warrant possible reconstruction.

For example, many people interviewed said that, "I solved things myself" and "we did not give importance to things that could not be overcome but, rather, on those that could" (female, 40 years old). Others noted that "if you wake up alone and you are aware of yourself . . . you do not restart daily life if you are always with others" (female, 46 years old). The need to move on and cope with disaster is not always a unanimous and communitarian process, especially during the early aftermath. Some people need to be alone, and it can be better not to force the necessity of living within a community all the time. There is some personal soul-searching to be done before coming back to a sort of daily life: ". . .you don't ever come back to daily life" (male, 41 years old). This feeling of loneliness should be respected by volunteers and other people close to them because, as mentioned earlier, emergency changes people deeply, and during this period people may behave in ways that sometimes remain difficult to explain and understand.

Because the Civil Protection Voluntary Service had just started, the Umbria earthquake was characterized by many experiences of personal and individual resilience: "I cheered myself up" (female, 40 years old); "what I could do I did" (female, 48 years old); "I am going on alone trying to be powerful. Then everyone reconstructed their life" (female, 41 years old); and "everyone has created something" (male, 41 years old). Individual resilience was present through the determination and stubbornness of some people: "in the end if you want something, you must do it"; "you weren't going to be overcome, you wanted to win" (female, 48 years old).

These attitudes highlight the presence of individual resilience that could be studied, not only from a psychological point of view but also from a sociological one, considering the importance of the primary and secondary socialization processes as the main topic for a deep understanding of sociological resilience. However, people affected by disaster also search for human and altruistic relationships. "I needed someone to help me. . . . My daughters needed help" (female, 48 years old); the reconstruction was possible "thanks to the help of many people" (female, 48 years old), and people's main worry was for relatives and parents: "I cried a lot because I was worried about my daughter" (female 2, 40 years old).

Civil protection volunteers and volunteers in general had an important symbolic role relating to the response to the disaster: "afterward we also had this safety net, someone was there for you" (female, 41 years old). It is proper that the volunteers and the Service are subjected to the attention of sociologists: "regarding the question of voluntary service. I think it has been the most beautiful thing of the earthquake" (female, 46 years old); regarding volunteers: "we have also welcomed them" (female, 48 years old).

Although many felt that "you start with a loss of hope, because really you think, 'there is no one to help me'" (female, 46 years old), the high degree of assistance that pervaded the experience of the Molise earthquake – "in general, everyone helped the others, even those who didn't really help, as such, helped with social organization" (male, 41 years old) – was not present during the experience of the Umbria earthquake. Some aspects of resilience also seem to be linked with the issue of gender, which is a basilar question for disaster study but has not really been considered for disaster resilience. "the women helped, the men were insular and anguished, they were not reactive" (female, 48 years old).

The mission of volunteers starts at a specific time after the initial behavior: "when you stop to think, it is terrible, you cannot face it" (female, 48 years old). The image of the civil protection volunteers was characterized by one interviewee as follows: "the civil protection volunteer is, however, a human, they do things, it is not enough to be grounded. . . . The difference between one team and another is down to the coordinator, she/he must see, overseeing . . . she/he was able to comprehend your need" (female, 48 years old). From this sentence arises the issue of leadership during a disaster, and its importance is underlined by the fact that not only is the leader's professionalism or level of technical competency important and fundamental but the personality of the coordinator or leader is more relevant – her/his ability to manage the feelings and needs of both the population and the volunteers themselves. Studies of this issue highlight the importance of organizational aspects, the leadership process itself, and the leader's identity (Murphy 2009). The influence of the leaders, and their personality during disaster management and life in a shelter camp or afterward, should be deepened for rethinking crisis and disaster management models in the future.

At the beginning of the mission, even if welcomed by the population, civil protection volunteers can run into disadvantaging opinions or behaviors. "There are people who do not comprehend the role of volunteers, above all the elderly . . . they are not able to identify with her/him" (female, 46 years old). This attitude is not specific to the Umbria earthquake; in the Abruzzo earthquake, someone described the civil protection volunteers as strangers: "those people, we can say, are being helped [by] the inhabitants themselves" (male, 68 years old), especially with resources and knowledge about the territory and infrastructure.

The mission of the civil protection volunteers was evaluated by the interviewees. "In my opinion it has been managed quite well" (male, 68 years old); "[these relationships] have given me a lot from a human point of view . . . a relationship that has changed my life" (female, 48 years old); "[they are a] friend of everyone" (male, 48 years old). However, "as everywhere else, this participation is decreasing. Before there was the passion to do it" (male, 48 years old).

People interviewed told me about their relationships with the volunteers and the help they gave: they "[looked] for a way that did the least harm possible" (female, 48 years old). This is important, especially for the strong need to respect the symbolic and traditional link with the territory and the homeland stricken by the earthquake. "Many people go away from the place, families with children are missing and people from outside came in, people who are not of the village . . . they are not people who care for the village" (female, 46 years old). This aspect is true more for the villages situated on the mountains and hills than in the city. In this context, from a sociological point of view, in part there is new thinking about the dual perspectives of the community and society, as argued by Toennies (1979/1887), which matches contemporary ideas about some features that characterized the relationships established in these contexts.

Another consideration is the importance of meaning and traditions attributed to a territory and homeland. The differences of strangers coming from far-away places can undermine the whole resilient process, which at that point the community affected by earthquake has barely started. In this context, importance also is given to the role of place and space as a facilitator of memory, both social and historical (Halbwachs 1987), which act as a fundamental resilient instrument for disseminating and informing youth and others about potential risks.

Relationships between the civil protection volunteers and the population affected by earthquake were meaningful. ". . .[Y]ou have established friendships which are maintained even up to today. We are happy and proud to have maintained these friendships" (female, 46 years old); "we are still in contact" (male, 68 years old). An important aspect about the relationships between the civil protection volunteers and the population is the continuity of voluntary service for a period after the emergency phase: "it is important that you remain afterward because the situation is like this for 3, 4 years. . . . Because until the real and concrete reconstruction of the village starts again, you need support" (female, 46 years old).

This represents a key sociological resilient issue and point of conflict among experts who work within crisis and disaster management. The common thought lies in the necessity of providing first aid, rescue, and response to basilar needs; many technical experts in the civil protection sector, however, believe that voluntary services must be present only during the impact and emergency phases. Instead, as previously suggested, the figure of the civil protection volunteer should remain for the whole period of reconstruction because "everything was a mosaic, in little pieces" (female, 48 years old). It is possible to rebuild the "mosaic" only through the intervention of many diverse groups, such as ordinary people, institutional personnel, civil protection authorities, and civil protection volunteers.

Trying to distribute and manage the few resources people have available within their own territory and what comes from outside is important. The issue of resources and their distribution is another key factor in terms of best practice within disaster management and the prevention of waste: "you found a lot of waste" (female, 41 years old). This situation is common, above all during the emergency and when there is a lack of response to primary needs.

It has been said that the disaster experience changes people, transforms them into someone else. It also influences social relationships: "beautiful friendships we had before the earthquake, maybe they were ruined because of these problems" (female, 46 years old). This is the core problem of a disaster and the reason why a disaster is a social disruption and critical event. Sometimes what a disaster destroys is not just houses and buildings but, above all, social relationships and people's equilibrium: "the fear and the tranquilizers have done the most harm" (female, 41 years old). Many people suffered from posttraumatic stress disorder, but during that time not much attention was given to the condition.

The aspects described here reveal the importance of sociological disaster resilience and the complex framework within which the issue has arisen.

8.3.3 Conclusion

It is not possible to say that, after 14 years, the Umbria earthquake underwent any sociological disaster resilience process, although the village of Nocera Umbra is still being reconstructed. It is not possible to understand what happened there because there is still a church and some historical buildings to construct. There have been problems reconstructing historical buildings as they were before the earthquake because they were made with ancient stones and it is difficult to reproduce them exactly. Another problem is that many families left, taking their children.

Nevertheless, as mentioned earlier, it is possible to recognize different dimensions of the disaster resilience process. "We must be aware of where we live, events such as these must teach, help many people" (female, 48years old). In terms of tradition of the homeland, memory about one's own territory can become future lessons for subsequent generations. "The important thing is that you recreate a place that you like" (female, 46 years old). The discussion about place for the Umbria earthquake, which is different from the outline of the life story, has concentrated attention on the homeland and village in the question of housing. The affected population had few illusions about their own houses and their reconstruction.

The circular process of helping is realized through the relationships between the civil protection volunteers and the population affected by the earthquake. "For this reason there aren't specific 'helpers'; in the end the helping has been from everyone" (male, 41 years old). Regarding the civil protection volunteers, "this deep friendship has remained . . . I would like to meet them again, but I do not remember their names" (female, 41 years old). The final aspect of this resilient relationship concerns the role of memory and its weaving that remains after everything: "they never forgot us, we never forgot them" (female, 48 years old).

A personal attitude of determination and individual resilience – "you need some guts to be able to remain" (female, 46 years old) – is a vital one that can be developed throughout life: "now maybe I am becoming stronger" (female, 40 years old). After the presentation of these paths to disaster resilience, a general conclusion about resilience as related to this earthquake is represented by the following statements: "we were able to be a community" (female, 48 years old); "we are used to the idea that, from a disgrace always comes something good" (male, 41 years old).

These two are the fundamental dimensions of discussion about disaster resilience. People identified themselves, not alone, but as part of a community, and this is pervasive for all locations: the mountains, the hills, and Foligno city. This communitarian attitude has many sociological implications for the disaster resilient process. One interviewee expressed this well:

> My heart was overwhelmed on the one hand, that was that period, but on the other hand I have had many rewards, much satisfaction. There is that hole that remains and doesn't fade; logically, other than that, I have many beautiful things. . . . I only hope that there will not be another earthquake. My hope for the future is always, in my opinion, that I will be more predisposed toward others . . . and be more open. Do not think that I don't feel good, I feel well and I have everything and I have my place, I mean, I feel good, I have everything, but if others who are close to me also feel good and have everything, I am happier. (Female, 46 years old)

8.4 Molise Earthquake in 2002

Discussion of the Molise earthquake should be framed because it is not completely a sociological discussion about what happened. Instead, because of the historical, social, and political circumstances, it is a short chronicle about some considerations of the general feelings that pervade my impressions of Molise society.

The Molise earthquake in 2002 can be remembered as the "children earthquake" because 27 children died, along with their teacher, in a school in San Giuliano di Puglia. In addition, two other people died in that earthquake. The death of the children (including the mayor of San Giuliano's daughter, who died in the school) was, and is even now, dramatic and important to understand the whole emergency and disaster management process.

In particular, this human loss caused the degeneration of relationships between the populations living in the villages close to each other and produced rivalry among different villages. The same rivalry exists during the distribution of the aid after earthquake because it seemed that all aid was concentrated in San Giuliano di Puglia and that many other villages were forgotten. For example, while San Giuliano di Puglia (a village with 500–600 inhabitants) has been completely rebuilt (including the construction of a university), Larino, another village stricken by the same earthquake, has still to be fully reconstructed (some has been rebuilt). During my staying in Larino, I came to believe that the main cause of all these problems is that, as mentioned earlier, the event created a concentration of external resources and relief aid from other regions of Italy toward only one village.

The ancient rivalries between the villages that were close to each other were present before the earthquake itself and enhanced conflicts and not collaborative relationships. In the following analysis, the rivalries and misunderstandings between these people are presented through the words of interviewees, in particular, an interview with a young woman.

Another element of my misunderstanding was that I was unable to get to that village using public transport. There are no buses that go to San Giuliano di Puglia or Casacalenda and there is only one train to Larino that runs twice each day. Furthermore, there is no connection between the villages. This reality is not just a simple question of mobility but is import to sociology fieldwork. In fact, the difficulties I had during those days was, for an "outsider" like me, a point of reflection about the influence that physical place and spatial organization have on sociality and the social relationships between people.

This aspect also is fundamental regarding the organization of relief aid, first aid, and the feelings of isolation experienced by the local inhabitants. Furthermore, the myth of a sunny and friendly Southern Italy was, in this instance, completely surpassed. It is important to understand better that many variables are involved in a social organization and it is not so simple to generalize.

However, it seems to me that social cohesion and solidarity are opposite, even if the context is a rural community: social cohesion, as Russell (1949) explained, and organic solidarity within a community, argued by Durkeheim (1893), do not seem to be present within these rural communities. The feeling can be distinguished by referring to two categories: us and the others; I experienced this when I was there.

As we will see later, these dynamics have influenced and oriented the disaster management and, above all, the displacement and reconstruction phases. As demonstrated in one of the interviews, an interviewee mentioned that there is a basilar jealousy between the people who had the possibility of reconstructing their houses and those who have been unable to do so.

I examined many other sociological and methodological considerations, which I explain in Chap. 10, because they specifically concern feelings of researcher, with practical implications for the research project itself, methodological notes, and sociological reflections.

For my research on the Molise earthquake, I interviewed four women aged 22, 35, 66, and 67 years old. The question of gender is always present in this analysis. In fact, with regard to the Molise earthquake, two online questionnaires were completed by men, but I collected life stories from four women. To explain this process, various theories might underlies these dynamics: on the one hand, the possible availability of digital devices and the few participants within the voluntary service who were women; on the other hand, the distrust and the suspiciousness the people had toward me as a researcher played an important role during the collection of these interviews, taking into account that three of them were collected in the municipal building in Casacalenda and only one in a private house. Furthermore, one woman arrived with her father and another with her husband. Reflections about this as well as their related implications for the research process are explained in Chap. 10.

8.4.1 Life Before the Earthquake and the Impact Phase

One of the most important categories that disaster sociologists need to know within their research object is normality and the routine timeline that characterize the life of ordinary people. According to the interviewees, "Our family was a very normal family" (female, 66 years old); "I had not free space" (female, 66 years old); and "I lived in the old town and it was nice because I was close to my grandmother, my cousins, my uncles" (female, 22 years old). And on the day of the earthquake, life was going on as usual: "I was 13 and we were celebrating Halloween at school" (female, 22 years old).

The earthquake changed everything – it became a turning point, and the feelings of the impact, physical as well as emotional, were described by the interviewees. "Some minutes before the earthquake, I felt unwell and I felt a tremble underfoot" (female, 66 years old); "the electricity pole was waving . . . the car was shaking" (female, 66 years old); the "asphalt smoked, no smell, dust everywhere" (female, 66 years old); and it was noisy "like a truck of stones" (female, 66 years old). These feelings seem to be universal during all earthquakes because of the features of this physical and natural occurrence.

The time after the impact was characterized by the first spontaneous aid and by the effort of giving sense and meaning to what had happened: "during the first night everyone was in the middle of the street" (female, 66 years old) and "all the neighbors were together and were talking to each other" (female, 66 years old). First aid came from neighbors, "as you can ask for help" (female, 35 years old).

A disorienting feeling was present: "I did not feel anything, because I was dancing so I was already on the move, my best friend came to me find me, otherwise I would have stayed there" (female, 22 years old). In this sentence one aspect of relief aid is represented; it was a methodological choice not to include spontaneous aid offered by parents, relatives, or friends but it is not uncommon, even if it requires adequate consideration as part of specific research programs.

Disorientation is also due to the lack of prevention and information about potential risk. "It's not that I remember so well because we were all caught in panic, . . . because we . . . they had never explained anything to us and before we did not know what we had to do" (female, 22 years old).

8.4.1.1 "The Old Town is Dead"

The Umbria earthquake made clear that the places and the houses of people are points of reference that orient life and its organization. In particular, the downtown area represents the core place where many public institutions, services, and shops are concentrated. It is the reason why experts talk about business continuity as an important factor, not only for private industries and infrastructures but also for general public services. After the impact of the earthquake people understood that, "the old town is dead" (female, 22 years old).

Individual houses were damaged as well: "The house was all quiet, we missed our place, our house, we worked for a long time on the house" (female, 66 years old); "I prefer to be hungry in my own house" (female, 66 years old). With the coming of new megacities and diverse concepts of cities, it is difficult understand this visceral affection, but it must be considered, especially during the displacement phase; they had to "leave their house, built with the efforts of [their] whole life, . . . the little things of the children, useless but very important for the emotions" (female, 66 years old). Because emotions are involved, time passes before people realize they need to leave: "your mind does not tell you to leave" (female, 66 years old).

The future management of earthquakes is based on the possibility of returning home: "we hope to go back as soon as possible, otherwise I would go away" (female, 66 years old); lack of this possibility causes the high mobility that has characterized the years after the earthquake, and it has increased this process, which may already have been present before the earthquake itself. People want to return home because "coming back home, you gain serenity and quiet" (female, 66 years old).

The question of house and place is a generational thought that is present among the elderly and the young: "an elderly person wants their house when they are sick" (female, 67 years old); "we never had a place to play" (female, 22 years old). Public administrations and the Civil Protection Service should understand these feelings and take them into account during disaster management.

This beautiful sentence represents the best argument: ". . .[I]f you do not feel safe in your own house, where are you safe?" (female, 66 years old). Safety is an "old" need of mankind, and even if everything changes in people's lives, it remains the first need to be responded to, in particular within a geographical area and a community potentially at risk.

8.4.2 The Image of the Civil Protection Volunteer and the Population: Help Received and Offered

Various social dynamics are present during the aftermath; during the Molise earthquake, the imperative was, "One thing is living it, another is watching it on the television" (female, 66 years old). Not all interviews were characterized by this strong differentiation between "us" (earthquake victims) and "others," the people who did not lived through this dramatic experience and therefore do not understand what it is like.

The disaster management during the Molise earthquake can be identified according to different points of view and considerations. Twenty-seven children died; this destroyed generational trust and institutional recognition, led to these families closing ranks on themselves, also and made it impossible to activate a reconciliation path and community resilience process. Children are the physical and symbolic ties among people in a community, and their deaths represented the end this and the impossibility of future generations and the ability to hand down historical and collective memories: "even the stones cry when they go there [the cemetery where the children are buried] . . . the thoughts were for the children" (female, 66 years old). In addition, the social cohesion among inhabitants of the villages was already damaged before the earthquake itself: "probably the village is not safer than before . . . it was also like this before the earthquake" (female, 35 years old). Another interviewee stated that, "the Larino people are . . . envious, bad I remember it was always thus, their mentality is dull, ancient about everything . . . we are a bit backward" (female, 22 years old).

The main lack of disaster management in this context was, as mentioned before, the absence of prevention, information, and communication of the potential risk; a warning system; and structured local civil protection organizations. "Local civil protection was not prepared, instead it was prepared by the other regions. . . . "Now the civil protection volunteers are prepared, but that year [2002] they didn't have any specific training, they were ordinary people just like us: (female, 66 years old). This lack was crucial not only for the relief-aid organizations and emergency management but also for the future and implications for reconstruction. In fact, people live with a sense of insecurity: "today, I am frightened to open the door . . . [it is] knocked on by unknown people" and "it is not as quiet as before" (female, 66 years old).

Sometimes relationships also change after a natural disaster the social: "before the earthquake we had good relationships with neighbors, after they were damaged" (female, 66 years old). Reconstruction often is confined to its technical aspects and does not concern the sociality and the human relationships present in a community: "they are still rebuilding it, for 5 years . . . it is the same country but it is divided, also . . . it is another mentality" (female, 22 years old); "as if I had changed the country" (female, 22 years old); "the earthquake has ruined everything, also the affections" (female, 67 years old).

This research has supposed from the beginning that the civil protection volunteers, local as well as from other regions (with other kinds of implications), probably could have an important role in the negotiation and recognition of what had happened to the population and in enhancing the resilience process, although they must be trained in the best manner possible. However, this seems to be not feasible in this context; in 2002, people did not recognize and know the civil protection volunteers and their activities. "We did not know that they existed and there was no Civil Protection Service, nothing of civil protection; after the earthquake they founded the Civil Protection Service" (female, 67 years old). Despite this, the civil protection volunteers "assisted us as much as they can" (female, 66 years old) and ". . . were good people, professional and human" (female, 67 years old). In addition, "the institutions came to look at us" (female, 66 years old).

In general, because of the external aid coming from other regions, in a context of welfare model of crisis and disaster management , such as that present in 2002 during the Molise earthquake, the feelings of the earthquake victims were oriented toward helplessness: "the day was useless" (female, 66 years old), and "we could do almost nothing" (female, 67 years old) because "we were looked after . . . they ask us what we wanted" (female, 66 years old). The attitude of the earthquake victims was sometimes characterized by "feel[ing] like doing nothing" (female, 66 years old).

Feelings of uselessness, the inability to take an active part in the emergency response, and the legitimation of a basilar role in the intervention was against the faith (as the earthquake was seen as related to external causes). This was the image of the region, which did not have the fundamental principles of prevention, preparedness, and emergency response. The aid came, for the most part, from the other regions and, the amount of damage compared to the amount of aid is not well correlated.

Furthermore, the issue of aid is related to the issue of the distribution of aid and the availability of resources. In particular, according to the words of the ordinary people, it seems that in San Giuliano di Puglia there was a concentration of aid: "in other villages [one of which is San Giuliano di Puglia] there was more presence" (female, 35 years old). In part an ancient rivalry among the villages that increased with the earthquake was confirmed by the availability of resources during the emergency response and reconstruction and by an unequal distribution of aid: "there were people who still had a home and came to eat at the tent city" (female, 22 years old).

However, the civil protection volunteers demonstrated their strategic role in a sociological resilience process: "with the first people of civil protection who came [from Lazio], we had contact, we were one big family, all together" (female, 22 years old); "they did useful things, necessary for everything, a friendship was created during a difficult time" (female, 67 years old). Civil protection volunteers were considered as "crucial in all," and "they did not want to move, they wanted to stay close to us" (female, 22 years old). They also are recognized with particular attention by those who had children: "they tried to play it down to the children" and when they helped "you did not have time to think neither negative nor positive" (female, 22 years old). In times of emergency the borders of trust and distrust change to facilitate a possible resilient process: "then, whatever, you had to trust everyone" (female, 22 years old).

Finally, as we will see in the following conclusion, the Molise earthquake is characterized by the high degree of novelty within the framework of sociological disaster resilience.

8.4.3 Conclusion

Writing a conclusion to the analysis of the life stories collected from those who lived through the Molise earthquake in 2002 is not a simple task because of many factors. I could not do a rhetorical analysis about the regions of Italy, but, sociologically speaking, the previous condition of the region stricken by the earthquake should be considered in terms of a framework analysis. As the comparison among all three earthquakes has demonstrated, it is not a question of the location of the earthquakes

(South Italy). Umbria is in the central area of Italy and even now people are still living in temporary housing, for example, in Valtopina. This aspect involves not only the geographical location of the earthquake but also its impact on the cultural context and institutional resources. The possibility of activating a regional Civil Protection Service for disaster management has been possible only according to the set of competencies, skills, and instruments tested in the time of peace. In addition, talking about earthquake prevention is not simply a discussion of engineering interventions or geological awareness and preparedness; it is also about preparing the people potentially at risk through institutional resources and specific services dedicated to these phenomena. Finally, in Italy, the issue of earthquakes, floods (such as the recent ones in the Liguria and Toscana regions) as well as natural disasters in general and their consequences on the population affected is unfortunately a never-ending question that afflicts all the aspects of postmodern life and its social organization: "life is not normal, I do not know but maybe it is the discontent that a useless year has passed"; "too many years have passed in this way, so that we were in a condition that a person [becomes depressed]" (female, 67 years old). It seems that no one is interested in the discontent and depression felt by the victims of the earthquake. Shops and other commercial activities have not reopened, and the passing of time makes this situation worse: "it is not the village that is changed, the services have changed in all the villages . . . the earthquake has intervened, but it is not related to this. . . . It concerns more of a personal and psychological level" (female, 67 years old).

Furthermore, "many people had gone away" (female, 35 years old), and "after 10 years I am still away from home" (female, 22 years old). The core issue of housing seems to undermine the people and their resilience and creates these feelings of discontent and depression, but the importance of housing in terms of individual, personal, and social identity is central. "I don't have the same enthusiasm as before" and "I do not recognize the house" (female, 67 years old). By "not recognize the house" she means that she does not recognize life now compared to that before the earthquake and does not have a mental place within which to collocate this dramatic experience. All things in the house are now located in other, temporary places, which are not her own house: "things that I do not recognize and I do not remember having" (female, 67 years old). Sociologically speaking, material things and objects determine our individual personality and the way others know us. For any individual, to lose everything and not remember having these things is quite like losing a piece of ourselves, our story, and our symbolic place in the world.

Those who experienced the Molise earthquake had to cope with the deep, sorrowful fact of the death of 27 children. The ambivalence of the earthquake and the resilience process are always present but, after all the research and its analysis, with this earthquake there existed a strong individual resilience: "a person does what she/he can" (female 67 years old). The most beautiful example of individual and familiar disaster resilience was the statement, "I have the feeling of the necessity to be pregnant, because you understand that life is brief" (female, 35 years old). Pregnancy has many symbolic and anthropological implications because it is the act of creation and the possibility for another new and, it is hoped, better life. This quote is gendered oriented because it was said by a woman in a particular stage of life. Although common, in the aftermath of an earthquake pregnancy assumes multidimensional features:

- Individual resilience for the woman and familiar resilience for her mate and the close community.
- The link between generations and historical and social memory.
- The best symbol of continuity and reconstruction against sorrow and pain.

Furthermore, pregnancy is the symbol of trust in life and in the social organization within which the new child will live.

Another dimension of disaster resilience is presented in terms of individual resilience: "I am very positive, so I always try to eliminate bad memories, bad thoughts" (female, 22 years old). The memories linked to and the stories told about the earthquake are not simple to collect: "that is, we really do not talk about the experience" (female, 22 years old), and this is demonstrated by practical behavior: "I am not informed. It is my choice, I have continued to live my life" (female, 22 years old).

The real thing that has determined this individual side of resilience is "knowing that you can do something to save yourself" (female, 22 years old), but the people who lived in Molise when the earthquake struck were certainly not prepared to cope with the earthquake and its consequences: "the mind is stopped in a time before the earthquake" (female, 66 years old).

8.5 The Abruzzo Earthquake in 2009

The Abruzzo earthquake in 2009 will be remembered as the L'Aquila earthquake. To understand better the disaster management at a geographical level, it should be said that L'Aquila is the capital city of the Abruzzo region and is divided into 19 hamlets, with one representative for each in the municipality of L'Aquila. This is an important issue with regard to emergency and disaster management and for the relief aid and its distribution. It is also a crucial aspect for the delicate issue of reconstruction and the distribution of resources (economical, infrastructural, and logistical).

After this earthquake, 308 people died; many of them were university students and young people, who were sleeping in the houses of older relatives or parents that night because for some days the earthquake tremors were becoming stronger and more worrisome. The number of deaths was too high to cope with.

Some days before the earthquake people had asked for information about the continuous tremors and were reassured by the local, regional, and national authorities: "in December [2008], during Christmas, these shakes continued, the earth did not stop moving. . . . By then we were used to it" (female, 52 years old). This is typical, causing a loss of trust in the institutions and authorities that should guarantee the safety of the population. Before this earthquake, as well as the other two earthquakes discussed earlier, no type of prevention was activated, even though L'Aquila is considered to be in a seismic area.

Eight people were interviewed about this earthquake:

- Male, 46 years old
- Female 1, 52 years old
- Male, 55 years old
- Female, 50 years old
- Female 2, 52 years old
- Male, 63 years old
- Female, 58 years old
- Female, 47 years old

It is necessary to point out that the following analysis looks at the phases of disaster but excludes the reconstruction phase because it is only just beginning.

8.5.1 Just Before and During the Impact of the Earthquake

It sometimes happens that ordinary people have the extraordinary power to describe a sociological and methodological question through the use of words that are disarming for the potential of representation and an evocation: "now what I am saying is influenced by the fact that we have suffered the earthquake" (male, 63 years old). The awareness demonstrated by this interviewee about storytelling and the method of telling one's life story with no intervention from the researcher can provoke some interesting methodological considerations about the biographical method of a life story. First, it is based on what people decided to tell; this assumption was discussed earlier. Second, as with the Umbria and Molise earthquakes, this natural disaster divides the life of the people affected by it into two different periods: before the earthquake and after the earthquake. Third, utilizing the life story as a methodological approach within the sociology of disaster allows the researcher to compare the timeline of the emergency with the lives of the people affected by it; this can be difficult but it could be interesting for future longitudinal studies about this. Furthermore, the biographical method and the disaster process are linked by the question of time and its passing. This could lead to some interesting research about the individual resilience process and the different moments of life itself; in fact, being affected by an earthquake when you are young compared to when you are older are completely different experiences. This is a fundamental difference also demonstrated by the analysis of the other earthquakes. Finally, many interviewees who lived through the L'Aquila earthquake expressed gratitude to me for allowing them to talk about what they suffered and giving them someone to listen to their story. I got the impression that for these people this represents a moment during which they could reflect quietly about the dramatic experience they lived through; however, sometimes people that did want not to talk about the moment of the impact: "it is not useful to tell what has been" (male, 55 years old).

All disasters and, in particular, the L'Aquila earthquake are characterized by the breaking of routines and the normality of life: "my life before the earthquake was a very normal life" (male, 55 years old); "my life was quiet and organized" (female 1, 52 years old); ". . .life was normal" (female 2, 52 years old); and "our life was quite regular" (male, 63 years old). During the moment of the impact all the previous certainties were broken and nothing was ever the same: "The vicissitudes of life change some situations" (male, 46 years old) "because the earthquake is a thing that is devastating" (female 1, 52 years old). The earthquake itself has a generational link with past experiences lived through by relatives or parents: "it is a thing you felt when you are children" (female 2, 52 years old).

The description of the impact featured physical and symbolical aspects: "when it started [it was] indescribable" (female, 58 years old); "it has been terrible" (female, 47 years old). This general feeling is concretized by various interviewees: "we were woken up by a strong noise" (female 1, 52 years old); "the noise of the gas in the pipes it was like a gust of wind; this shocked me" (female, 50 years old); "you hear the walls moving" (female, 58 years old); and "you felt the house turn around you, everything moved around" (female, 58 years old).

The disorientation was always present. "We did not understand immediately what was happening" (male, 55years old), ". . .at that moment I did not understand what really had happened" (female, 50 years old). There is a sort of incredulity among people who have lived through an earthquake: "earthquakes have never provoked me to panic" (female, 50 years old). This feeling of incredulity is deeply correlated with the normality of life and the routine organization of life itself. This is a strong element of personal and, in some ways, communitarian vulnerability, which should be the subject of new studies because of its importance in determining an approximate level of vulnerability and the consequential possibility of intervention and enhancing resilient attitude toward potential risks present within a geographical area.

During these moments people were lucid enough to "immediately [notice] that something was not right" (female, 58 years old), and after the first impact recognize that "your first thoughts are the worst" (female, 58 years old). This feeling is made possible according to different aspects of the situation itself, including the lack of resources: "we didn't have a car" (female 2, 52 years old) and "we did not know where to go" (female, 47 years old).

The lack of personal and individual resources in this context is the core element of the possibility that one person survives or responds better to the emergency. In addition, other types of resources, such as infrastructural, logistical, or organizational ones, have completely collapsed as a consequence of the impact, and for this reason it is not possible to trust in the continuity of social organization because it is stricken by the earthquake in the same way. It could be interesting to analyze the different kinds of vulnerability and their effects when they occur one after another.

It is also important to comprehend when this lack of resources is caused by a personal or individual lack or, instead, when it is caused by the actions (or lack of action) of public services and institutions: "we were used to it, but above all you were desensitized" (female, 50 years old), probably because "prevention is a word that does not exist in this nation" (female, 50 years old). "If they would say something, we could prepare for it, but if the authority said there was nothing to worry about, we believed them and so we have suffered much more as a result" (female 1, 52 years old).

The management of this earthquake was lacking from the first phase of prevention (we will see later the complete absence of training courses about earthquakes) and preparedness, which consists of early warnings and best practices for when an earthquake occurs. None of these actions were done before the impact and unfortunately 308 people died, many houses were damaged, and some villages, such as Onna, were completely destroyed.

This process recalls the FAKKEL model presented by Clausen (1992); he theorized a symbolic and social connection with a tie between the authorities and the population as victims. This model is important for a sociological approach to a disaster because it focuses attention on the dynamics between these two subjects during the disaster and the implications in terms of communication, information, trust, cohesion, and the possibility of rebuilding the tie that is broken through the intervention of the disaster and the inability of the authorities to safeguard the population.

In this way it is also possible to try to realize a disaster resilient process, starting with the analysis of risk of the communication systems and the organization of training courses. Out of a deterministic approach, one must be aware that even with the creation of training courses for the population, not all damage will be avoided, but the Japanese organization of prevention teaches us that better preparation and organization is possible. So, what is important is the organization of training and a communication program for people living in at-risk areas.

After the impact "we were there waiting for it to end" (female 1, 52 years old) and "I could not find the dog" (female, 47 years old). "The first thing I did was get my mother-in-law and my dog" (female 2, 52 years old) – obviously the first thoughts were for relatives and parents: "the rush to go and see the others [in my] family" (female 1, 52 years old).

Once people were able to leave their homes, they found that "outside was worse than inside" (female, 58 years old), and "there was nobody there, it was a desert and you did not understand what you must do and there was a strong smell of gas" (female 1, 52 years old) – "we were like zombies" (female 1, 52 years old).

Before the full emergency phase, the relief aid arrived. "The relief aid came early, and this seemed, to me, suspicious in that, maybe, they were alerted before" (female 1, 52 years old). If this were be true, it would confirm the statement and explain that they authorities expected the disaster but did nothing to create prevention and preparedness involving the population potentially at risk.

8.5.2 *After the Emergency*

These stories allow us to understand that, after the first moments of disorientation and not comprehending what happened, the worst period for people affected by this earthquake – and natural disasters in general – is after the impact and the beginning of the real emergency because of the deep necessity of sense- and meaning-making that occurs.

This process of sense- and meaning-making could be a basilar individual and social process for disaster resilience and, for this reason, civil protection volunteers could be the link of trust and disaster resilience between institutions and the population. In the Umbria and Molise earthquakes it does not seem very linear; this was caused by many factors that will be summarized in the conclusion.

However, during an emergency and its aftermath, people have diverse reactions: "I had a strange reaction, that is, I burst into incredible tears" (female 1, 52 years old); "when the emergency phase had just passed, one says, 'oh, well, we're all alive,' but then you begin to think that there is no home, there is no work, because I did not work before the earthquake; someone said to me, 'but what happens now, what can I do?'" (male, 55 years old). After the impact, people had to decide what to do in this situation, and the model of relief aid in the L'Aquila (Abruzzo) earthquake was the building and organization of tent cities, which remained for 9 months. In the beginning, however, some people who had their own tents or caravans organized a spontaneous camp just to give first aid to each other: "everyone tried to go to a place where they had no risk" (male, 55 years old). Another interviewee stated:

> From the place we were [a spontaneous camp] we started to see them taking away the first rubble and they piled it up near us and then they brought a machine, I do not know exactly what it was, that loaded up the things and from those piles. You saw the pieces of the life of the people; clothes, photos, documents, also pictures of children, and this thing does harm, this thing does harm. It was quite difficult for us go there and see this rubble, we just heard the machine that worked, just the noises, during this week; I must say that it was hard." (Female 1, 52 years old)

"Pieces of the life of the people" is the best image that was collected during this interview. It represents the confirmation of routine and normality broken by the earthquake and the irreparable damage to life and the deep sense of family, safety, and future expectations. Because earthquakes, and natural disasters in general, are synonymous with destruction and the end of all future projects, the resilience process is important to enable people to cope with and face up to these events in an attempt to guarantee a minimum of continuity and trust in the future.

As always, relationships established during the aftermath have the ambivalence typical of this situation, unlike the Umbria and Molise earthquakes, which used two different models of crisis and disaster management. In L'Aquila the model of response was based on the temporary housing in the tent cities until some new temporary houses, called New Town, were built and people could be moved there. Staying for a long time in a tent with other people (the tents sometimes could give shelter to seven or eight people) created some difficulties: "living together in the camp was not always easy" (female 1, 52 years old), and "I was definitely more comfortable at home" (male, 46 years old).

In particular, the distribution of resources, as usual, created some problems. "At first they gave things out without control, then, of course, there were some who took more than others" (female, 47 years old). "They gave things out to many people . . . they took a lot of aid" (female 2, 52 years old). "It was annoying, that was all, and they were good at managing it, knowing how to contain it, then some little unpleasant episodes happened, but it's over now" (male, 55 years old).

In this situation it is difficult to think about a general model for the distribution of resources based on the response to fundamental needs, which are universal in all natural disasters. Standardized instruments cannot be used; instead a more flexible tool needs to be designed based on the specific emergency. This step could represent an enhancement of institutional resilience belonging to the Civil Protection Service and, according to the international literature, better distribution of resources could help with the disaster resilience process and its future development.

It should be clear that creating a rivalry among people affected by an earthquake during the distribution of resources, and considering people who do not need aid in the same way, seems to be a failure of the public institutions and the symbolic trust that people have in them. In fact, the distinction between those who must be helped and those who do not need help must be clear and made public to allow relief aid and the local resilience process to function well.

In spite of all the inconveniences experienced by the earthquake victims within the tent cities, there have also been good relationships. "In general I have always had good relations with people" (male, 46 years old), and, "for some people, going away from the tents, it has been traumatic, because, above all, in the little camps, some ties were created" (female, 50 years old). Living for a long period in a tent, however, is not the best solution for the elderly: "here, the elderly were treated the worst" (female, 50 years old); "she was perceived as a nuisance, she survived . . . but the shock was too much for her" (female, 58 years old).

In this situation, not only the elderly, even if they are recognized as the more vulnerable social groups in this case, but also adults in general had many problems: "the use of psychotropic drugs and antidepressants trebled" (female, 50 years old), and there were "clear symptoms of stress after the earthquake" (male, 46 years old). Regarding this argument, we can consider research done by the University of Camerino, which unfortunately confirms this trend. In my opinion, this also confirms that a possible social and communitarian resilience process for the L'Aquila earthquake has not yet occurred.

8.5.2.1 The Image of the Civil Protection Volunteers and the Population: Help Received and Offered

During the emergency phase, the civil protection volunteers had a crucial role in the relief aid process and giving assistance to the population: "they helped until they almost physically collapsed" (male, 46 years old), and "they were very good, they immediately organized everything . . . above all, because the dog must sleep with us" (female 2, 52 years old). The "civil protection volunteers were very human, they understood us (female 1, 52 years old). "At that moment I was so grateful to them because it was the same for them because, in practice, nobody knew what had happened. It was a sick period of time, however; there was gratitude to the people who came, many volunteers came" (male, 55 years old). "You must appreciate the act, that despite everything, they were here . . . in general they were people to admire, to appreciate" (male, 46 years old).

Although this image of the civil protection volunteers as people interested in the well-being of others and, above all, the earthquake victims, the feelings for these people were mixed. "I hated all of them" because "sometimes there was some conflicts for the showers and, in fact, some people left the camps in desperation" (female 50 years old).

Only eight life stories were collected from survivors of this earthquake and analysed, but many other stories were collected that, for many reasons, I decided not to use. Many of these stories identify the civil protection volunteers as strangers who came from other regions and sometimes did not comprehend the real needs of the people affected by the earthquakes, The civil protection volunteers who came from Basilicata, where some years ago there was a strong earthquake, were welcomed: "they had already lived through an earthquake and so they knew what it was" (male, 55 years old). However, there was also the opposite side of this consideration: "[the volunteers] do not know what it means, the sacrifices of a life of generations" (female, 58 years old). This clarifies the impossibility of meaning-making by the civil protection volunteers who live in a different situation: "today everything is painful . . . there has been a twisting of space and time" (female, 50 years old). In fact, disaster as a social process changes the time and space coordinates and the perception of them.

One woman notes that, "as time passed things diminished, that is, [the volunteers] were less competent, but good all the same . . . during the last period they gave us nothing" (female 2, 52 years old). This is an important aspect correlated to the maintenance of the tasks and competencies attributed to the civil protection volunteers. As we have seen, the volunteer in general has many reasons to go on with or stop voluntary activities, and it is necessary to understand and make explicit this normal feeling during the training courses for the new volunteers. In this way it may be possible to overcome burnout and the other feelings of frustration and a sense of impotence.

However, the feelings of the population affected by earthquake toward the civil protection volunteers often were characterized by collaboration and reciprocal tolerance: "well, that depends a bit on you interacting with them, but if you interact with them, they were available" (female, 47 years old), and "instead we tried to make friends" (female 1, 52 years old). It is an effort during the aftermath of a disaster at many different levels – psychological, emotional, personal – and it would be better if the civil protection volunteers themselves could be aware of all these individual and social dynamics.

8.5.2.2 The Places and the Houses Stricken by the Earthquake

When an earthquake occurs, the landscapes and, obviously, the cities and villages are stricken by its destructive energy: "the geography of city has changed . . . now it is another city" (male, 46 years old). In particular, places are of interest in disaster resilience on different levels"

- Before the emergency: create training and preparedness activities for the Civil Protection Service and volunteers as well as for the population at risk
- During the emergency: must take into account the disposition of cities and villages, coordinate the first aid, and consider the feelings of the inhabitants for their places, cities, and villages.

- After the impact: respond to the emergency and to the needs of the people affected by the earthquake and specifically take into account the feelings and the perceptions of the population for the place and their belonging to that place: "I come from L'Aquila and I want to remain in L'Aquila and many people must leave and go far away . . . that is, I was born in L'Aquila and I stay in L'Aquila, are we becoming like boxes? I do not think it is right, I do not think it is correct" (female 2, 52 years old). The sense of belonging and the willingness of people to stay where they grew up requires respect from all the institutions and agencies involved in the disaster management process; they should realize that "when it was a red zone, attempts were made, and I felt the need to go into the house to find something" (female, 58 years old).

The place and its use have a crucial role in the localization of tent cities and temporary houses after the emergency period and during the decision about where the temporary houses were to be placed. "Many people came from here and we came all from the same area, the old Monticchio, because that area has been damaged and so we are from all the same area, so they are neighbors and people from the same area" (female, 58 years old). After this period there were other problems: "I didn't have the courage to face the walls of the house again" (male, 63 years old). After the earthquake there were diverse housing solutions, such as the tent cities where families waited for temporary houses, private housing, or a hotel in L'Aquila or on the coast. Some "were located outside" (male, 46 years old), and "those who accepted have left" (female 2, 52 years old).

All these solutions, mostly waiting for new houses, created various problems. "The family is all scattered, I mean some live in one place, some in another" (female, 50 years old). "You cannot meet with each other, because there are no places where you can meet" (female 50 years old). In particular this seems to be one of the most important obstacles to the social reconstruction of L'Aquila and its surroundings.

An interesting process to be considered is the coming "home" to a temporary house given by the Civil Protection Department and Ministry of the Interior after many months spent in a tent: "going into a closed room was very nice" (male, 46 years old), but "in the house we don't feel as if we are in our house" (female 1, 52 years old). In fact, the housing solution is a temporary situation, and precarious feelings dominate the life of the earthquake victim: "in the new house we have acquired a little bit of normality, although I must say it felt a little cold, you do not feel free, also because, I repeat, this is not a home" (male, 55 years old).

Sociologically speaking, the house represents the social and communitarian life of a person, and losing a house is like losing a part of one's own identity: "then the demolition of house has started . . . and so no house, it isn't there, it is a desert and over the rubble, the grass does not grow. I think that they built there again, considering that they have demolished the house, but the problem is that nothing moves and the silence has shocked us" (female 1, 52 years old). Assisting with the demolition of one's own house is a dramatic experience that marks people forever. It is the physical loss of place that means family, safety, and private life; life in a civil protection camp and months in a tent mean the sharing of all daily activities, even those more private.

Among all this pain, some people have had the strength to be happy for others living in a better situation: "at the beginning it was beautiful to see the people coming back home, even from outside the area" (female 1, 52 years old). The displacement phase is not only constituted by logistical and technical aspects, which must be organized; there are many individual and social aspects that must also be considered to facilitate the next phase of the reconstruction. During informal chats, ordinary people in L'Aquila told me that the decision to displace not only older people but also families to the coast was not the right decision to maintain the core traditional and social memory of the place itself and to favor the economic and social reconstruction of the city and villages.

8.5.2.3 Disaster Resilient Process

The first thing one should know about the Abruzzo earthquake is that little reconstruction has been done yet, so it is difficult to have a discussion about the reconstruction phase. One ordinary person interviewed said that, in his opinion, the reconstruction phase will require more than 15–20 years. I personally visited L'Aquila and its surroundings twice, in May and June 2011, and I was shocked by the state of the downtown and its surroundings. The first thing that came to mind was, "How can they think that any sort of reconstruction is possible in these conditions?" In fact, the necessity of a double kind of reconstruction – both social and physical through the rebuilding of houses and public places stricken by the earthquake – had already been argued. Those two types of reconstruction are interrelated, and it is not possible to distinguish them in a clear way.

Although this critical situation got worse day by day, a beautiful example of disaster resilience from a sociological point of view was found in the personal attitude of finding something positive among all the sorrow: "there were also many positives things, which were not there before" (male, 46 years old).

There are many other examples of disaster resilience that identify the multidimensionality of this social attitude. One is the individual side of disaster resilience and familiar resilience in the aftermath: "we personally are helped by ourselves" (female 1, 52 years old); "I must solve mine, my own problems" (female 2, 52 years old); "after that, I thought about how to react, how to fix us" (male, 55 years old). Familiar resilience has had a crucial role for many people after the earthquake: "by this fact [his niece's death] the whole family is ruined" (male, 63 years old); "I didn't became crazy because, thank God, I have my family close to me" (male, 63 years old). In this case the family reconfirms its strong role of support and help for all its members. Another dimension of sociological disaster resilience is the presence or absence of social relationships external to one's own family: }there is the fact that there was V., he gave all of us the strength to cope" (female, 58 years old). The presence of another person who needed care was the factor of resilience for a whole family and the other people who shared the tent. The prosocial attitude demonstrated by the person providing care can be considered sociologically oriented and resilient oriented: the strength to cope and go on is given by another person external to the family and their members.

In this situation the idea about others also quickly changes: “it is nice to find a known face” (female 1, 52 years old), and “we began to think with a more open mind toward others” (male, 55 years old). Unfortunately, sometimes there was not the possibility to experience this resilience: “everything has degenerated” (male, 46 years old), and there is a “different awareness” (male, 46 years old). Sometimes death changed everything: “only one of my neighbors survived” (male, 46 years old). In general, the perception of others is constituted by suspicion: “people have changed and people are getting worse, they are more selfish” (male, 46 years old); “the friendships that I had before are almost all gone” (female, 47 years old).

Even with this negative experience, the ambivalence within a disaster context is present, as always: “then many things have changed, because this experience has scarred me a lot. This experience, at least as far as I am concerned, helped me to have relationships with people” (male, 55 years old). Another man said that, “you spent your time doing things that you previously did not” (male, 46 years old). The aspect of social resilience is present within the stories of the people interviewed: “it’s not that I did it alone, we all worked on it” (male, 63 years old).

As I said before, in a geographical context such as L’Aquila and its surroundings, it is very difficult to maintain social relationships because there were no public spaces in which to meet together and the displacement of parents, relatives and friends created problems for the mobility of these people: “it is difficult to maintain relationships at a distance” (male, 46 years old). This must be a point of reflection for disaster and emergency management because displacement is a crucial question to be considered in accordance with many factors, such as geographical distribution, mobility, intervention with landscapes, sociality, and availability of sharing places

The final dimension of resilience analyzed for this earthquake is an institutional one, above all, the proposal of training courses for the population potentially at risk: “the training courses are important” (male, 46 years old); “I think the training would be indispensable” (female 1, 52 years old). Training seems to be necessary, and the population at risk must be informed of and trained for the event for which they are at risk. The population should have the cognitive and material instruments to face the risk and cope with the disaster. For the L’Aquila earthquake in 2009, however, it seems that the situation was the complete opposite: “in L’Aquila there was absolutely no information” (male, 55 years old); “we do not know anything, because in reality we are able to know it 2 days later” (male, 63 years old). Training courses for the population are necessary to try and avoid disaster – “they knew what they had to do but, instead, probably that was the fate” (female, 58 years old) – and make possible both intervention against pure fate and the participation of more people in the prevention process: “that is, if a very strong earthquake happens, we are powerless, we cannot do anything, we can only suffer it” (female 1, 52 years old).

8.5.3 Conclusion

After 3 years, the Abruzzo earthquake has reached the reconstruction phase, although as I said before, there are no material signs of this occurring. According to my personal experience, people’s desire to rebuild and go on with their life is there;

however, in spite of this, I noted that many people have left the area and others are deeply emotionally broken.

The people there have various attitudes. Some are resilient: "[I'm] looking ahead" (male, 46 years old) and "the only way to survive in this situation is to participate in the things that are happening; I do not believe that there is another way to survive" (female, 50 years old); whereas some are not: "I've given up everything for now, I do nothing, I'm here and I wait" (female, 47 years old) and "I did not want to participate in anything" (female, 47 years old).

It is true that for the past 5 years, "this life is an emergency life" (female, 50 years old). People are stuck in that period: "I always try not think about it again" (female 2, 52 years old). They have no trust in the institutional agencies and administrations: "we hope for aid but we do not believe in them" (male, 63 years old). It seems that the lack created after the impact of the earthquake has degenerated the relationships between the public administrations and the population affected by the earthquake: "they gave us a car, but did not give us the fuel to make it go" (male, 55 years old).

It is impossible for the population to rebuild the cities and villages alone, without external aid from the public sector and specific departments, regions, municipalities: "that is, we try to move; however, is not that we move so well" (male, 63 years old). A sense of loneliness and frustration is clearly present: "here, however, there's plenty, we have everything, but we have nothing" (female, 58 years old); "this has not been the earthquake of building, but of reconstruction" (female, 50 years old), referring to New Town and the lack of respect for the places and the locations before the earthquake.

Finally, the following quote is from an interview and summarizes all the aspects of a possible and desirable disaster resilience process, such as all the sorrow, pain, sense of belonging, and loyalty to one's own place:

> Surely the house has to be removed as it is not possible to have it shored up. It was one of the first houses shored up, inside and out, and it's all underpinned throughout, with iron all around. I go there every day, I try to go every day, because I have a dog down there, because it cannot be brought here, but one goes there just to go there to see. When we were at the tent camp, I came from work, we took the car, loaded my mother who still has not understood all this, and we went to the park in front of the house and then again later on in the evening. Many times we ate in the car, outside the house, every time we brought something back, some tomatoes, anything because we did not like to go to the tent to eat and, no, we did not like it, because there was everything, but one wanted to feel as if nothing had happened: 'let's go take a vacation there,' and then we go [back] to the camp. We did it often, recharging ourselves, and then returned to the camp, we returned to the camp and tried to live normally. (Female, 58 years old)

8.6 Final Conclusion

This research was presented earlier as explorative and not comparative, and for this reason three fieldworks were chosen. I do not want to lead an analysis comparing the diverse findings that were collected singularly. However, I present here some general conclusions that concern all three earthquakes and what was defined as the disaster resilient process from a sociological perspective.

The analysis of the Umbria earthquake (1997) suggested that there was a community resilience used to face the disaster. In fact, the findings seem to confirm this suggestion: a core of feelings was found among the people interviewed, who came from different locations such as the mountains, the hills, and the city. It seems that this kind of attitude was pervasive among the population in general and related to the communitarian tradition within which they live. A core agency, such as the family, was an useful "social agency" used to maintain contact with others. Taking care of children is a link with the whole community, as is the effort to keep with their own territory and houses.

The resilient dimensions from a sociological perspective were based on the high level of social trust and social cohesion, which allowed the community resilience response to the earthquake. In this case only the possibility of sharing the dramatic experience they lived through and strength, both individual as well as social, guaranteed the reconstruction of the community and buildings.

Regarding the situation in Valtopina, where to date people still live in temporary houses and not in the "hot zone," there were difficulties in contacting these people, and the political polemic covered the specific vulnerability of these people and the institutional agencies. One thing is clear: political rivalry and controversy must be separated if the aim is real resilient reconstruction. In fact, politics had demonstrated that it is not efficacious and is not useful in coping with a disaster. One thing that can enhance institutional resilience and improve the implications of it for disaster victims separating technical and management practices from political ones: the mixed situation does not to make for a resilient response to a disaster.

Regarding the Molise earthquake, the dimensions of disaster resilience are the individual and familiar ones, which seem more present in the aftermath and within the reconstruction phase here. People tried to find housing solutions using private resources such as private temporary housing, displacement, or leaving.

In Molise, not everything is a consequence of the earthquake, but it is clear that the situation mentioned above in Valtopina, characterized by rivalry and disintegration among the communities and villages, influenced the aftermath of the earthquake itself. This is a typical social vulnerability that stops the processes of reconstruction and resilient response. People did what they could, but the lack of prevention and preparedness was too great to allow a communitarian resilient process.

Finally, for the Abruzzo earthquake, there have been many theories about when the reconstruction phase will start and when people will see the effects of disaster management and political management on their life courses. However, in my opinion, there are two different discourses here. One concerns L'Aquila city: if buildings are not reconstructed there, nothing will change because too many people have been displaced and others have left because of the lack of mobility and jobs. Villages (excluding Onna, which was completely destroyed), on the other hand, have the right potential and social resources to take an active part during the reconstruction phase and implement a resilient disaster process: the future is now, within the decisions that are made now.

The final consideration about the disaster resilient process from a sociological point of view is the identification of categories that can be used to try to classify this research experience. Sociological resilience processes, such as primary and secondary socialization, are influenced and oriented by the vulnerability of the system and the population itself, as well as the use of available resources. The social identity of a singular person and her/his prosocial attitudes and behaviors allow disaster resilience to be developed using social and human capital as basilar instruments within a specific ecological framework, such as the environment in which a natural disaster has taken place.

A social resilient identity is based on some assumptions that are common to all three earthquakes (sometimes only one or two of these dimensions are present, and sometimes they are mixed):

- A traditional and generational way of understanding and perceiving fear, troubles, disasters.
- A normative social identity – "I must do it" – where the norms and social communitarian values are so strong in the life of a person that they orient a resilient response to a disaster.
- Caregiver: "I must be strong for my children, parents, relatives." This is a traditional familiar attitude, but it also has important social implications for the family members involved.
- A defeatist attitude, typical of people who wait for a solution from external agencies or entities. This social identity has a lower level of social resilience because it is more individually oriented.

It is possible that all these social attitudes are generated by a primary and secondary socialization process, and it is possible to enhance a more useful disaster resilient response through training and courses for prevention and preparedness that are dedicated to the whole population potentially at risk.

Chapter 9
Conclusion: Final Proposal

9.1 Toward a Relational Approach for Disaster Resilience Planning

The aim of this final proposal is to present a general conclusion after the collection of all the data and information from the semistructured interviews with civil protection experts, the online questionnaire completed by civil protection volunteers, and the life stories of the earthquake victims. The final results can be understood within the theoretical framework of sociological theories and the previous definition of disaster resilience from a sociological perspective.

In this context, different patterns of disaster planning and disaster management are shown, with practical consideration for those used and interpreted during our fieldwork in areas affected by the three earthquakes in Italy. These patterns were analyzed through general dimensions of social life and the presence or absence of them during specific disaster planning. Three mixed models of disaster planning as they related to the three earthquakes in Italy were considered.

After this theoretical and methodological presentation, a different model for disaster planning was considered based on a resilient and relational approach from a sociological perspective. The assumption and the future challenge of disaster planning is to consider resilience in the preventive and preparedness phase, as well as considering civil protection volunteers together with other volunteers as "resilient agents" for a resilient disaster process.

This research, even if it is complex, could be considered as an important starting point for future research and training programs in the fieldwork of disaster resilience and its comprehension. Referring to the theoretical background that influenced this research, as previously illustrated, some sociological theories were fundamental to elaborating the theoretical context within which it was possible to orient this analysis. According to the different sociological orientations and the definition of disaster resilience from a sociological perspective, we were able to analyze and interpret a disaster resilience model for each of the Italian earthquakes considered here.

B. Lucini, *Disaster Resilience from a Sociological Perspective*, Humanitarian Solutions in the 21st Century, DOI 10.1007/978-3-319-04738-6_9,

Table 9.1 Disaster resilience planning and management patterns/models

Disaster planning and management phases	Disaster resilience operative categories and their features/strategies					
	Social	Cultural	Organizational and political	Communicative	Economic	Environmental
1. Prevention and preparedness						
2. Response						
3. Displacement and recovery						

This final proposal considers and analyzes the whole process of the three models or patterns of disaster resilience planning during the three earthquakes in Italy: data collection and analysis through semistructured interviews with experts in the civil protection system, online questionnaires completed by civil protection volunteers, and life stories by ordinary people affected by earthquake.

At the end of this chapter we propose a general model for disaster resilience planning and training activities in the field of disaster management and response. It is necessary to specify that these models have no claim of generality, but they should be a starting point for reflection on fundamental topics of social relevance, such as disaster resilience and the actions taken by different people and agencies involved in crisis and disaster management.

Furthermore, specifically regarding the interviews collected from ordinary people, we need to remember that we have already explained the decision to interview only Italian people. It is believed that the cultural dimension, which belongs to migration, should be considered as a challenge for future research in the field of disaster resilience.

The analysis of the three earthquakes in Italy contemplates the use of the definition of disaster resilience and the patterns proposed in the previous theoretical elaboration. Table 9.1 shows the possible combinations between the presence or absence of the resilient categories explained in Chap. 3 and their related features, dimensions, strategies, and disaster planning phases such as prevention and preparedness, response, displacement, and recovery. The different combinations of these elements can recognize previous patterns of disaster planning and management: conflicting, narrative, collaborative, coordinative, supportive, and resigned (Table 9.1). Specifically, the patterns of disaster planning can be explained by their general features.

9.2 Patterns of Disaster Planning

The main aspect of conflicting patterns is the social disorder and confusion caused by some decisions made by disaster planning groups and the gap between the organizational culture typical of the institutions aiming at disaster management and the population affected by the disaster. This conflicting aspects causes an interruption in terms of socialization and the related disaster resilience process; the flow of communication appears fragmentary and incoherent in the context in which the disasters have taken place.

Instead, a narrative pattern is characterized by the metaphorical and rhetorical level of communication and information sharing among all social actors involved in the disaster management process. The message of risk and disaster communication is aimed not only at coordinating the disaster management process but also at informing other people and the public about what happened in an attempt to identify and underline different positions of all the social actors involved (e.g., confronting the Molise earthquake and the death of the children during it is such a communicative process within a narrative pattern).

A collaborative pattern is based on the assumption of an organizational and operative culture that is typical of the Civil Protection Service and its related disaster management processes. The collaboration style allows all people involved in the disaster management process to participate, focusing on the identification of a communicative pattern and sharing cultural meaning belonging to all the people and agencies involved. Related to this pattern is the coordinative model, which is based on an assumption of coordination and shared information and a communicative process.

The coordination pattern is deeply related to the organizational cultures of the different agencies involved in the disaster management process. Attention is focused on the dynamics of leadership and the negotiation activities of the members of the organizations. In particular, it is related to the institutional and administrative mechanisms of the civil protection organizations and based on the specific goals and objectives of disaster management.

In contrast, a supportive pattern is based on proactive, helpful attitudes and social cohesion principles, typical of voluntary agencies, that can facilitate the displacement and recovery phases. Volunteers can be considered a fundamental and strategic link between people affected by disasters and those responsible for disaster management. This pattern is considered the resigned model of disaster planning and management based on the impossibility of the people involved to create proactive disaster management dynamics and improve their life conditions after the disaster. It is characterized by a static and inactive dynamic, which is not fruitful in terms of the disaster resilience process. Within this pattern, there a circular logic is elaborated among all the people involved that is not proactively oriented; for instance, abandoning a city and villages stricken by an earthquake is a common action that influences the possibility of rebuilding the cities themselves and the communities stricken by disaster.

According to the discussion about different patterns, above, we need to consider that disaster planning can be constituted by various patterns and their related characteristics within a specific phase of disaster planning. The following takes into account some important features that emerged from the analysis of the three earthquakes in Italy.

9.2.1 *Disaster Planning Patterns of the Umbria Earthquake*

Regarding the Umbria earthquake, because of its specific features the disaster planning model and its related phases can be defined as collaborative, participant, and supportive patterns. During the prevention and preparedness phase, the operative categories, their features, and strategies included the following:

- Social strategies: Because of the organization and environment, characterized by closed communities, social cohesion/solidarity was present among the population before the earthquake.
- Cultural strategies: We can say that at the time of the earthquake a shared culture of seismic risk did not exist and that no type of training activity was proposed before the earthquake itself.
- Organizational and political strategies: Before the Umbria earthquake, the Civil Protection Voluntary Service was in its infancy and permitted the involvement of other voluntary services; this was one of the most important social and organizational aspects.
- Environmental strategies: Attachment to place was present within the population and can be evaluated through the traditions and habits related to the location.
- Communicative strategies: There was a lack of crisis communication with and training of the population potentially at risk.

During the response phase, the operative categories, their features, and strategies included the following:

- Social strategies: Ties of trust, solidarity, and social cohesion were created and activated among the people affected by the earthquake and the volunteers who intervened during and after the emergency.
- Cultural strategies: The cultural identification process was evident, with the first distinction among different types of disaster subculture: the subculture of people affected by the earthquake, the subculture of volunteers involved in disaster management, the subculture of institutions aimed at coping with disasters, and the subculture of mass media.
- Organizational and political strategies: The process of participation of different social actors and agencies was possible despite normal conflicts in this situation. Social actions and interactions were based on the general features of collaboration and support, allowing the possibility of effectively responding to the crisis that occurred.

Within these categories, there was the presence of the influence of the typology and organizations of local, provincial, regional, and national voluntary services.

- Economic strategies: There were some difficulties in the distribution of the resources made available by volunteers and diverse agencies. This seems to be a critical point during all response phases, as in the other earthquakes.
- Environmental strategies: A sense of community and place attachment allowed most people to decide to reconstruct in the same place as before the earthquake.

- Communication strategies: The flow of communication between institutional agencies and citizens' committees were organized through the recognition of a representative of the people, who could be a resilient communication link between the institutions and the citizens themselves. This communicative and relational strategy has been a means of guaranteeing and maintaining social order, provided that the distance between the institutional agencies and the citizens does not become unbridgeable after the social change that always and inevitably results from an earthquake.

During the displacement and recovery phases, the operative categories, their features, and strategies included the following:

- Social strategies: The presence of volunteers and their activities were characterized by helpful and supportive actions for the people affected by the earthquake, allowing them to travel a path together and face the displacement phase in a hopeful context.
- Cultural strategies: The population in general was able to interpret their atrocious experiences and share common meaning- and sense-making processes regarding their situation and the possibility of rebuilding their towns.
- Organizational and political strategies: During the Umbria earthquake, the Civil Protection Voluntary Service was not as well structured and organized as it is now, but all types of voluntary services and organizations where present in the field of the Third Sector.
- Economic strategies: The economic resources to rebuild were negotiated between the population and local, provincial, and regional institutional agencies, and this negotiation process allowed the uses of funding to be checked.
- Environmental strategies: The displacement phase of the Umbria earthquake was characterized by the different steps that people accepted to rebuild in the same place struck by earthquake. This was represented by different steps in housing, moving from tents to containers and from these to wooden, temporary houses.

An important choice by the population and public agencies was the decision to rebuild homes and public buildings in the same place where they were before the earthquake. This has allowed for the creation of a social and historical memory of the community affected by the earthquake.

- Communicative strategies: Shared and useful communication flows were present between the population, public institutions, and other agencies; these can be enhanced through the role of volunteers as facilitators in the social and communicative processes.

9.2.2 Disaster Planning Patterns of the Molise Earthquake

Regarding the Molise earthquake, because of its specific features, the disaster planning model and its related phases can be defined by conflicting, narrative, and resigned patterns.

During the prevention and preparedness phase, the operative categories, their features, and strategies included the following:

- Social and cultural strategies: Preexisting conditions of rivalry and the fragmentation of communities, closed to each other, were present. It seems that conflicts and competitions among the different communities have a historical and cultural background. This situation did not allow the development of strong social cohesion and solidarity, which could be readily activated during the emergency.
- Organizational and political strategies: No training activities were developed by these communities for the population potentially at risk. Furthermore, the Molise earthquake occurred in 2002, and at that time there was still not a structured and organized local civil protection organization within the municipalities considered in this research.
- Environmental strategies: There was less knowledge about the characteristics of the location and its potential risk.
- Communicative strategies: No risk communication training or activities were developed before the earthquake.

During the response phase, the operative categories, their features, and strategies included the following:

- Social strategies and cultural strategies: The pre-existing conditions of fragmentation and little social cohesion did not facilitate response strategies. Furthermore, people affected by the earthquake were not used to seismic risk and did not have the possibility to interpret and share a common meaning and sense of the earthquake. In particular, the death of children as a result of the earthquake had created a social and community divide that, as of 2011 (the year of this research), had not yet been bridged.
- Organizational and political strategies: The territorial area and its institutional organizations did not facilitate the National Civil Protection Service to cope and respond to the crisis that had occurred. Also, within the municipalities struck by the earthquake (those considered in this research), there was no local civil protection association. For this reason, much aid was provided by other regions of Italy or the rest of the world.

In this phase, the organization of relief aid was difficult because of the preexisting conditions of community fragmentation and because the typical roles and competencies attributed to the public officers of the Civil Protection Service were not sufficiently recognized by the population.

- Economic strategies: The fundamental economic aspect is that the aid came from other regions of Italy and the rest of the world and was perceived as not equally distributed among the communities and municipalities stricken by the earthquake.
- Environmental strategies: Place identity and attachment processes were evident because of the different social identities and the interactions of the people who helped during this phase.

- Communicative strategies: The attention of the communication process was focused on the death of the children and the sorrow felt by their families.

This is the reason to consider this model as narrative: the communication model was based on a metaphorical and communicative level to make the public aware of this tragedy.

During the displacement and recovery phase, the operative categories, their features, and strategies included the following:

- Social and cultural strategies: Family played a fundamental role in the displacement and recovery phase. In particular, many people were sheltered by their relatives, parents, and friends. What must be understood is that the possibility of creating a common basis from which all communities can interpret the dramatic experience, for sense and meaning making, disappeared (if it existed at all) because of the little social cohesion that existed among those communities and the prevalence of a familiar response to disaster.
- Organizational and political strategies: In this phase some problems of interaction between the population and the institutions were present. In particular, the problems were related to the possibility of access to economic resources to rebuild houses damaged by earthquake.
- Economic strategies: Regarding the use of economic resources, some people used their own or public funding to rebuild their houses, and fewer economic resources were used to rebuild shops or other commercial buildings.
- Environmental strategies: Many people affected by the earthquake were displaced to the houses of their parents, relatives, or friends. Other people were displaced to tents erected by the National Civil Protection Service or temporary houses.

It should be considered that the recovery phase was an element of important social change because of the permanent displacement of people at some distance from their homes before the earthquake. Statistical data and some interviews underlined this aspect, leaving many municipalities struck by earthquake now inhabited by older and retired people.

- Communicative strategies: The communication process was characterized by the same fragmentation and social division that were important aspects during the whole disaster process. In particular, this aspect did not facilitate the recovery process or, especially, the social construction of the experience of the tragedy.

9.2.3 Disaster Planning Patterns of the Abruzzo Earthquake

The L'Aquila earthquake disaster planning model and its related phases can be defined by conflicting, coordinative, and participative patterns because of its specific features.

During the prevention and preparedness phase, the operative categories, their features, and strategies included the following:

- Social strategies: Social cohesion and civil participation among communities and important stakeholders who can be supportive in cases of crises or disasters were present.
- Cultural strategies: There was a shared and social memory about the social identity of the people, especially in L'Aquila, although there was not a specific subculture of risk in terms of a general and a seismic risk.
- Organizational and political strategies: Many nonprofit organizations and voluntary associations were present and were useful during the response phase. Furthermore, a structured and organized Civil Protection Service was present at local, provincial, and regional levels because it had evolved and improvement its management of crises and disasters.
- Environmental strategies: People were aware of the risk some months before the earthquake, but this did not allow a specific subculture of risk and its relationship to the environmental context to be elaborated or interpreted.
- Communicative strategies: There were no risk communication or training activities for the population potentially at risk.

During the response phase, the operative categories, their features, and strategies included the following:

- Social strategies: A general trust and community relationships, collaboration among diverse Civil Protection organizations and associations, a stakeholder who allowed a coordinative and collaboration process between the population affected by the earthquake and those who were responsible for the crisis and emergency response all were present.
- Cultural strategies: Negotiation and collaboration process were present between different subcultures of risk and emergency, such as the population, civil protection volunteers, public institutions, and voluntary agencies.
- Organizational and political strategies: The response phase after the L'Aquila earthquake was characterized by a fundamental coordination between all the civil protection organizations and volunteers at national, regional, provincial, and local levels. This phase also was characterized by some conflicting aspects between the population and civil protection organizations and volunteers, especially those who came from other regions in Italy.
- Economic strategies: As shown earlier for the other two earthquakes, from an economic point of view the real problem during this phase was the distribution of economic resources and primary necessities, which caused a social inequality that influenced the following phase of disaster management and the possibility of re-creating a sense of community.
- Environmental strategies: The collapse of the whole city of L'Aquila and its surroundings was perceived by people as the collapse of their social and community organizations. Specifically, the earthquake destroyed all the public offices and institutions, considering that L'Aquila is the capital of Abruzzo region. This

aspect oriented and influenced the community's sense of place and place attachment.

- Communicative strategies: During this phase, the flow of communication was coordinated by civil protection agencies, and there was an effort to create a link between the institutions responsible for crisis and disaster management and the population affected by earthquake. This coordinative aspect was not always present because there were gaps due to technical difficulties and problems as a consequence of the earthquake.

During the displacement and recovery phase, the operative categories, their features, and strategies included the following:

- Social strategies: People were driven by altruistic and proactive behaviors, and relationships between the population and volunteers were characterized by solidarity and social cohesion, even if there were some problems with the civil protection volunteers who came from other regions and with the immigrant social groups affected by the earthquake.
- Cultural strategies: Some cultural skills were used to face the disaster, but there was a lack of a common process of sense- and meaning-making about the tragedy.
- Organizational and political strategies: Displacement and recovery related to the Abruzzo earthquake was a critical issue because of the decision to leave people in tents or other temporary housing for a long period of time (up to 9 months) to wait for the so-called New Town, which included new houses built in another place and not located near the city or its surroundings. At social, cultural, and economic levels, this decision had important consequences for the life of many people, their families, and the community in general. It influenced and shaped the process of reconstruction and the possibility of returning to a "normal life."
- Economic strategies: The economy and business activities of L'Aquila and its surroundings was wrecked by the damage and the choice of displacement, as previously mentioned.
- Environmental strategies: The time and the modality used for building New Town and other temporary housing created a distance between the population and the place where they lived. This aspect influenced the sense of community and place attachment that was experienced, resulting in a feeling that nothing could be improved or changed.
- Communicative strategies: The flow of communication followed a coordination pattern and sometimes was characterized by a gap between institutional agencies and the population affected by earthquake. The fragmentation of information about the displacement and recovery process created a sense of confusion and neglect in terms of the necessity of creating a link between the community affected by earthquake and the institutions and agencies responsible for disaster management.

9.2.4 The Relational Pattern

The previous analysis of the disaster planning patterns used in the three Italian earthquakes and its typical patterns show some best practices and worst practices, which was elaborated during the management of these disasters.

According to the theoretical background and sociological framework, a diverse pattern can be presented for future disaster planning methodology that is able to respond to and achieve a resilient disaster plan for future crises and disasters: the relational pattern.

According to the typical features identified earlier and the phases of disaster planning, which include disaster resilience dynamics, we are able to identify and propose a relational disaster resilience plan that is based on social relationships and individual and social actions aimed at coping with crises and disasters. The focus on relationships (excluding reference to network analysis) allows us to consider fundamental social attitudes of solidarity, social cohesion, and altruism (Dynes 1994) during disaster planning as well as their related dynamics.

Furthermore, the role of the communication process within disaster planning should be considered through resilience characteristics in terms of coherence of the message, robustness of the channel, and the cultural and organizational subculture of addressees and those who send the messages. Risk and prevention communication should be improved in the preventive and preparedness phases to create a common and resilient subculture among the different social groups potentially at risk.

9.2.5 Resilience Strategies

A different point of view is represented by the possibility of communicating and publishing not only safer behaviors in cases of crisis and their impact but also resilience strategies that can be learned during the socialization processes and through risk communication programs.

Indeed, we previously assumed that risk is the product of vulnerable and resilient elements and aspects of a system potentially at risk. The fundamental assumption is that we are not only able to *be* resilient, but we *are* resilient. In this sense, risk communication during the prevention phase and the creation of a common and shared meaning concerning the crisis and disaster social process can define the capacity of the population affected by disasters and those responsible for disaster planning and management to respond in a resilient way (Lombardi 2005).

The circularity of communication and information is fundamental to creating a common relational resilient framework and promoting and sharing of social and cultural dimensions. Furthermore, training activities and communication programs are important aspects in developing trust, ties, and social cohesion between the population potentially at risk, local voluntary associations, and institutional agencies.

Specifically, during the past 10 years, an organized and structured Civil Protection Voluntary Service had allowed for the recognition of the possibility for disaster planning actions focused on social relationships and resilience as a socialization process at individual, social, and cultural levels. In particular, we need shared cultural and symbolic dimensions to identify a local community's sense and tradition in terms of risk, resilience, crisis, and disaster to be able to influence the future dynamics of disaster management, allowing the participation of the population in the elaboration of a disaster plan that is socially and culturally oriented. A relational disaster plan based on the final aim of improving resilience should consider all latent and evident social and cultural dimensions related to the systems potentially at risk.

In summary, we show some best practices for resilience and relational disaster planning in terms of practical tools and strategies according to the diverse phases of disaster planning. In the prevention and preparedness phase we must:

- Recognize and support the role of "resilience agents" played by civil protection volunteers and other volunteers
- Improve risk communication and safer behaviors of all members of the voluntary agencies that could be involved when crises occur to identify other stakeholders and not only the civil protection volunteers
- Improve resilience dynamics for risk communication and allow access to shared information about potential risk for all the various social groups present in a society in an attempt to enhance social cohesion and inclusion
- Organize training activities for children in schools, identifying them as "social agents" in terms of transgenerational dynamics of familial and social resilience actions
- Encourage environmental awareness about physical features of living places
- Elaborate a common and shared disaster resilience subculture among all social actors (e.g., the population, public institutions, voluntary services, the infrastructural system)
- Promote the sharing of information about resilience to improve the sense of community and active participation in disaster response

During the response phase we must:

- Explore and better understand the distributive dynamics of aid, primary needs, and economic resources, which seem to be fundamental elements, to determine social inclusion and socialization processes that are oriented around resiliency
- Recognize the role of civil protection volunteers as "resilient agents" and their specific attitudes of proactive behavior, altruism, and solidarity to activate a resilient response, including as many people as possible in the construction of the disaster management process
- Coordinate the flow of communication among all social actors, identifying the resilient features that each communication should have
- Recognize and better understand the specific disaster-resilient subculture typical of each of the voluntary organizations or other institutional organizations responsible for coping with disasters, according to their specific elements such as roles, competencies, leadership, and negotiation processes

During the displacement and recovery phase we must:

- Reconsider displacement strategies through relational and resilient patterns to support and maintain a sense of place and place attachment, allowing that the people affected by an earthquake can be supported in their community (obviously only when it is possible according to technical evaluation of the buildings and their damage).

When reconsidering the choice made during the Umbria earthquake and the different steps of the recovery phase, we notice that this decision made possible a sustained sense of community and increased social cohesion and solidarity actions that remained after the earthquake itself.

It was shown that the modality of displacement and recovery influenced in a strong way the resilient socialization process and the possibility of rebuilding the communities and cities stricken by earthquake. During this phase, we should not forget the importance of the civil protection volunteers and their presence. In general, volunteers are to intervene during the emergency phase, but it seems to be important to reconsider the role of support and helping after the emergency phase.

According to this, the role played by the local civil protection volunteers is basilar to sustaining the population after the emergency. During this phase, it is important to do the following:

- Try to provide and support specific programs for shared cultural and historical memories oriented to resilient socialization processes in the community.
- If possible, involve people in the organization of tents or other temporary housing to activate their own resilient process and make them active in the recovery phase.
- Focus attention on resilient communication flows and strategies of communication between the population and the institutions responsible for the rebuilding policies.
- Recognize the different resilient subcultures, with reference to place attachment and social legacies.

What has been proposed are general strategies and tools that need to be adequately considered within the social and organizational systems. Disaster planning and management through a sociological perspective and resilience approach and according to our complex and multicultural societies will be a future challenge within disaster studies.

9.3 Conclusion

Economic and political crises almost everywhere in the world mean of new era of change in cultural, economic, political, and social approaches to available resources. The promotion of disaster resilience from a sociological perspective takes into consideration the importance of being aware of our links to cope with and face disasters and crises in the best way possible. It makes it possibile to enhance and develop our individual resilience, and in some cases our own reaction to a critical situation can be a pleasant surprise.

It is best not to forget that disaster resilience is synonymous with democracy, that is, when people are able to respond on their own and use the resources available in their communities and societies. Disaster resilience also is involved in social organizations through the aspects of social cohesion, social control, and social conflicts. In fact, this research has shown that disaster resilience is not always or only positively oriented; as the German tradition of sociology of disaster has demonstrated, during disasters and crises social conflicts as well as the need for social control are present.

I have discovered that the difference among social cohesion and conflicts is the presence or absence of disaster resilience in all its dimensions is constituted by the presence of death. Although a situation such as the Umbria earthquake may be dramatic and grievous because of the loss of houses and places there were few deaths, when deaths are higher, as in the Molise and Abruzzo earthquakes, everyone suffers from the lack of linkages and ties of trust among the community: when children die, we lose a link with our own historical, collective, and social memories and everything reminds us of the importance of safety and security issues within a democratic context and the importance of being prepared for an emergency.

Balance among all these sociological aspects and a deep respect for witnesses of natural disasters or those caused by human actions can make possible a better response to a critical situation and enhance disaster resilience at different levels through the creation of new and better ties of trust, respect, and social solidarity.

Finally, I would say that this was not simply a sociological trip through "important" arguments. Personally, it has been a trip for me to discover my personal and individual resilience as well as my social relationships of trust and solidarity in the midst of the doubts, troubles, and difficulties of normal life.

Chapter 10
Methodological Note

Chapter 10 describes the decisional process within the methodology of social science to collect, in the best way possible, interesting, innovative, and useful data and information. For this reason, and because of the variety of social groups and their specific features considered within this research, this chapter is based on the necessity of using multiple methods, with specific attention on the main characteristics of the arguments studied.

I decided to explore the Civil Protection Voluntary Service and its dimensions using semistructured interviews with civil protection experts; an online questionnaire for all civil protection volunteers at a national level (it was the only way to reach most of them); and life stories of the earthquake victims, taking into account an ethnobiographical perspective. The limits of this methodological approach and the future challenges for social researches also were considered. At the end of this reflection, there is a general consideration of the fundamental principles of ethics in disaster and social applied research.

10.1 Introduction

The topic of this research has presented some difficulties from the beginning. In fact, disaster resilience from a sociological perspective linked with natural disasters and, in particular, with earthquakes is a different area of study within the theoretical approach of social sciences and, above all, of sociology. It has been a challenge for future developments in the fields of crisis and disaster management and disaster resilience planning.

There were some problems with the theoretical definition of sociological disaster resilience within a natural disaster scenario. All other authors defined resilience as an ability or capacity from many diverse perspectives. Instead, I theorize and suppose that disaster resilience could also be related to sociological features.

B. Lucini, *Disaster Resilience from a Sociological Perspective*, Humanitarian Solutions in the 21st Century, DOI 10.1007/978-3-319-04738-6_10,

The methodological question also has been a troubling issue throughout the whole research process (Stallings 2002). In the beginning, after explaining the theoretical framework and one possible definition of disaster resilience and choosing the natural disasters to be studied – the three earthquakes in Italy – I started to think about how to explore the ideas, and it was a troubled path. Attention was focused on two social groups that are, in my opinion, the two most interesting in a disaster resilient process from a sociological perspective: civil protection volunteers and the population affected by the earthquake. These social groups show different characteristics that seem to be fundamental within a discussion of disaster relief from a sociological perspective. Because of the complexity of the argument and the typical features of each social group, I decided to use different methodological approaches and instruments (Corbetta 1999), which are discussed in this chapter.

10.2 The Use of Diverse Methodological Instruments

As mentioned just above, because of the complexity and fragmentation typical of this argument, I decided to use multiple methodological approaches and their instruments. This was not a methodological exercise or an "experiment" but a necessity because of the practical organization of the arguments considered.

The first step was to reflect on how to interview civil protection volunteers. The organization of the Italian civil protection system is such that when an emergency occurs all forces and civil protection organizations at local, provincial, regional, and central levels intervene, depending on the degree of damage. Therefore it was necessary to interview all volunteers (or as many as possible): For this reason I chose to do an online questionnaire.

Before the online questionnaire was created, the content and format were decided upon. After an analysis of the literature on voluntary services from a sociological and psychological perspective, the following issues were included:

- Prosocial attitudes and behaviors
- Motivations to become volunteers, in particular civil protection volunteers
- The organization of civil protection with which volunteers are involved
- Experiences of three earthquakes
- The changing voluntary service experience

Even from previous experiences with civil protection volunteers, I did not know the specifics of their organizations and activity, so I decided to interview experts of and those involved in the civil protection system. These interviews were semistructured and were conducted with a specific outline that included almost the same issues used to create the questionnaire. The characteristics used to identify and select the experts to be interviewed were the same as those used by Tremblay (1983) and presented by Palumbo and Garbarino (2006):

- Position or role within the expert community
- Deep knowledge about the topic

- Available to collaborate
- Dialectical capacity
- Impartiality

After identifying the experts based on the above-mentioned features and performing the interviews, I recognized that there was a limitation to these interviews: the concentration of experts from the Lombardia region, where traditionally the question of the Civil Protection Voluntary Service is more developed and has more economic resources. In this context, attention focused on that during the construction of questionnaire.

Other limitations can be found within the interviews themselves. In fact, regarding the institution within which an expert works, the language and the arguments were very different from each other. In this context, I noticed that some people being interviewed had problems telling me about the real situation of civil protection volunteers within their organizations, and the language used was more general and evasive. Sometimes people asked me to turn off the recorder when telling me confidential information.

Another observation on this point was the sensibility of the interviewee's point of views related to their role and leadership positions within their organizations. In particular, as their professional level increased there was a sort of compliance of their ideas with those of their institutional affiliation. Other experts involved in provincial and local civil protection organizations who were interviewed expressed ideas that differed from those of their institutional affiliations; for instance, some difficulties, problems, and failures in the field of civil protection activities were identified. In general, however, the interview setting was useful for collecting a lot of interesting information that was used both for this research and the creation of the questionnaire.

A practical issue concerns the time needed to complete interviews with eight experts: 3 months, starting in January 2011 and finishing in March 2011. This timeline seems to be quite normal.

10.2.1 The Creation of the Online Questionnaire

The creation of the online questionnaire followed the theoretical issues that were deepened by the interviews with the civil protection experts.

After a primary version of the questionnaire was created, it was piloted using nine civil protection volunteers who were different in terms of age, sex, educational background, profession, and affiliated civil protection organization. This pilot testing provided some useful suggestions used to improve the online questionnaire; specifically, the questions about the type of civil protection organization and the leadership within the civil protection organization were changed. A second set of tests was sufficient to proceed with uploading the online questionnaire.

To facilitate completion, clear and simple language was used; the use of ambivalent, double meaning, evasive, overlong, and academic questions and strong, negative words were avoided. At the same time, the answer possibilities were limited where possible. In particular, the sequence of questions started with general experience and going deeply into the specific situations of the three earthquakes in Italy.

As usual for online research instruments, the online version of the questionnaire has both advantages and limitations. Advantages include:

- The ability to interview many civil protection volunteers from the whole national territory, which was a priority
- Low cost
- Short time required to complete the questionnaire (maximum of 15 min)
- Facilitating digital instruments to complete the questionnaire
- Anonymity (Palumbo and Garbarino 2006)
- No influence by the researcher
- Noninvasive research instrument

The limitations included the following:

- The personal decision of the volunteer to participate in the survey (or not)
- The personal choices regarding which questions to answer
- The problem of digital devices and the availability, or not, of technological instruments
- The written language of a self-completed questionnaire allows no possibility of explanation by the interviewer
- The questionnaire must be short and not complex
- There is no ability to control the process of completion of the questionnaire
- During the analysis phase there is no ability to generalize the findings because they are not related to a representative sampling. However, this limitation is not appropriate for this questionnaire because the main aim of this research process is the exploration of social actions and dynamics within a social context, such as natural disasters, and so the generalization of findings is not theoretical or methodological need

For these reasons, this form of questionnaire used in this context was the most appropriate methodological instrument for this research project, even if the limitations of the online questionnaire and its choice as a methodological instrument (due to the inclusion of volunteers from institutional and administrative organizations) did not allow another kind of sampling (because of the absence of a list of civil protection volunteers belonging to municipalities or local groups or provincial or regional associations).

10.3 The Access to the Three Fieldworks

It was previously noted that the methodological approach of this research regarding the population's experience of disaster was based on the methodological proposal by Bertaux (1998) and his ethnosociological perspective on life story.

For this reason, some methodological aspects belong, even if not directly, to the ethnographic approach. In particular these include the fieldworks themselves, access to the fieldworks, negotiation practices used to collect interviews, and, in general, being with people who were affected by an earthquake.

The epistemological approach within which lies this methodological approach is based on the assumptions of emic and etic points of view: "An emic perspective is one that reflects the insider's or research participant's point of view, whereas an etic perspective is one that echoes the outsider's or researcher's point of view. [. . .] Finding a relationship between emic and etic perspectives is not simply a matter of balance, but rather these two ways of seeing are synthesised to explain particular human phenomena against a broader canvas" (Madden 2010).

Emic and etic are two perspectives that reflect diverse storytelling about the same arguments but with different cultural and cognitive points of view: "Emics and etics have nothing whatsoever to do with ontological issues; the ontological status of any event, entity or process in the empirical world remains unchanged, whether that event, entity or process is described in emic or etic terms . . . it is our understanding of the phenomena, not the phenomena themselves, that is either emic or etic" (Lett 1990, cited in Nigris 2003).

Although this research conducted was in Italy, my own birthplace and culture, the argument of earthquakes and earthquake victims was unknown to me because I have never experienced an earthquake myself; I think this gap represents and explains the difficulties I had during my access to the fieldworks and collecting interviews. What was interesting was that the difference did not concern the cultural frameworks of the researcher and ordinary people but regarded a human experience.

For this reason, I think that one of the most important things during the methodological path of collecting life stories for such a sensitive issue is being with people. In fact, as Madden (2010) said, ". . . being with people in ethnographic research is not a simple matter of being in an ordinary sense; it is not some form of unstructured hanging out with people. While the aim of being with people is to approximate as closely as possible the feeling or sensibility of everyday sociality between the ethnographer and the participants, ethnographic hanging out is also saturated with instrumentality."

I agree with Madden (2010) on this point because, as he said, being with people is not a simple matter of closeness: even if I was not interested in "real" ethnographic research or collecting interviews when I visited the field, I stayed there for some weeks and, through the use of sociological observation and help received from some kindly people, was able to go to unreachable places. I lived some days in the aftermath of the disaster, especially that of the L'Aquila earthquake, where the situation after 3 years is the same as it was immediately after the disaster.

Being with people and listening to their impressions, ideas, and experiences – even if not within a research context – is a deep human experience. It is equally important in the research process with regard to ethics, but there must be a balance between the feelings of solidarity and closeness and the necessary distance for the research and the researcher's point of view.

> [B]eing with people in an ethnographic context is therefore a partial immersion, albeit a sufficiently deep and simulacrum of what it's like to "walk a mile in their shoes". It is from this perspective "close, but not too close" that ethnographers attempt to build reliable portraits of the human groups they work with. Being close allows for the ethnographic authority of "being there" to be parlayed into the text (the emic perspective), while remaining "not too close" allows for the authority of the critical expert to be present in the text (the etic perspective). The "correct" form of being, that which finds a balance between closeness and distance, is required to give a reliable and critical account and to produce a more rounded form of ethnographic authority. (Madden 2010)

In my opinion, this balance has been the most difficult thing to achieve within my research process, especially while interviewing ordinary people affected by the earthquakes. It is difficult to stay with people who have lost everything. In particular regarding the L'Aquila earthquake, personally I do not know how reconstruction can be possible in such a situation but must maintain the "right" emotional and cognitive equilibrium to be able to collect the stories.

With regard to access to the three fieldworks, I define fieldworks in a way that is quite similar to the definition elaborated by Madden (2010): "So, an ethnographic field is not equivalent to a simple geographic or social space, nor is it a simple mental construct of the ethnographer, but it does require both these elements. It is the synthesis of concrete space and investigative space that defines the ethnographic field and gives it its reason for being – it exists to describe, to interrogate, to question, to problematize, to theorise and to attempt to solve questions about the human condition."

I have accepted the idea that it would be a synthesis of concrete and investigative space; according to my proposal it is also the social space where social and human relationships take place; the concept of social milieu elaborated by Schutz (1932) characterized the studying of natural disasters by sociological perspectives.

My first access to the field was made possible through the help of the following gatekeepers: In Umbria, an employer in the Foligno municipality gave me names of another three people to contact, each in a different location: one in the mountains, one in the hills, and one in the city. Regarding the context of the mountains and the city, as mentioned previously, I interviewed the gatekeepers themselves as well as other people.

In Molise the matter was more complex because I had different ways to access and various gatekeepers, and finally I failed the real task in which I was interested. In fact, in March (2 months before the period of the interviews), I tried to reach by phone and e mail the mayors of the main municipalities stricken by the earthquake; in some cases, I did not receive any answer or reply. However, I received interest from mayors in San Giuliano di Puglia, Casacalenda, and Larino. The secretary of the mayor of San Giuliano di Puglia told me that there would be no problems with the interviews and that I only needed to provide them with the number of people I wanted to talk with: four was about right. The mayor of Casacalenda responded to me with the same availability and assured me that I was allowed to go to the municipality to interview people whom he had previously contacted. The mayor of Larino gave me the number of the civil protection office in the municipality and, from there, an employee gave me a name of an interviewee. There were some problems with access in Molise that I have difficulty explaining and comprehending.

I and the major of San Giuliano di Puglia agreed on the days for the interviews and his secretary told me that everything was confirmed, but 2 weeks before my arrival I received a telephone call from the secretary, who told me that there were problems with the days set aside for the interviews and that I needed to talk with the mayor for more information: I was not able to contact him; I received only evasive replies and no one told me what had happened. Because they agreed to participate and be involved, I assumed they understood the aim of the research and my role within the project; even though I explained everything in a way that seemed clear to me, it probably was not clear to them.

In Casacalenda, I had the suspicion that my presence was not welcome and felt distant all the time I was there. Although the mayor of Casacalenda had assured me that he had found four people available for an interview (he told me that he would be out of the office during that week but that his secretary had the names of the interviewees), when I arrived, nobody in the office knew anything about me, my research, or the interviewees. I therefore had no way of contacting the interviewees to confirm our meetings; the only thing I could do was wait for them and relying on them to remember to meet me. Three people came for the interviews, but they occurred on a different day than was previously arranged.

The situation in Larino was better and I had no problems with the interviewee.

In Abruzzo I had two sets of interviews at two different times. The first time I received the name of the gatekeeper from an expert I had interviewed in Milan and I had no problem meeting them. It was the same for the second set of interviews; in this situation, I had received the names of two gatekeepers from an expert I had interviewed in Milan.

As in Umbria, I had no difficulty accessing the interviewees in Abruzzo. They were available to go with me around the city and the villages and I received a lot of interesting information during those visits. I was able to walk a mile in their shoes (Madden 2010), and I am thankful for all I learned; it was one of the best experiences I have ever had.

10.4 The Life Stories of Ordinary People

The interviews had some particularities belonging to the fieldworks themselves. The interviews collected in Umbria were characterized by stories of an experience that does not following a chronological time line, but, in general, were divided into three parts: before the earthquake, during the temporary housing solutions, and their changes during the reconstruction phase.

The interviews occurred in a quiet and welcoming place in the interviewee's homes. In the last two interviews, the interviewees were a married couple; there was some confusion between them and they tried to help each other to remember better what had happened. During the interviews, I was relaxed and interested in what they were telling me; because I had used the outline of the interviews many times before I could concentrate on other interesting issues.

The situation in Molise was different; I interviewed only four people because of the difficulty of access and the misunderstanding between myself and the mayor. Three interviews took place inside the municipality building, and it was not the best place to collect interviews: there was no one else there so it was not a confusing location, but the limiting institutional context did have an effect. Furthermore, one interviewee came with her father and her 2-year-old child; the child's presence sometimes required us to stop the interview.

I must confess that to me the Molise earthquake was a distant experience characterized by the invisible distance and unlinked way of understanding. It was not possible for me to walk a mile in their shoes (Madden 2010) because too many differences were present and it was not possible to move beyond them. Even now I still do not understand the reasons for this: I asked the interviewees for their availability and if someone had refused I would have asked elsewhere. But what happened there was the almost total exclusion of my presence; I was considered a stranger and they did not seem to understand the legitimacy of a researcher being there. Perhaps I had a bad access point and, again, maybe the explanation of my research and my role was not clear, but what remains with me as meaningless is that I used the same behavior and techniques as I did with the other two fieldworks. One interview, however, took place in someone's house, and it was the most relaxing interview I had in Molise. This points out that the physical context influences the ability to tell about a dramatic experience such as an earthquake.

In Abruzzo, the situation was more complex because I had interviews in different places: two within the space of a civil protection association and all the others in their homes. Of all the places I had gone to collect interviews, in L'Aquila the experience was really touching because I was interviewing many people who had experienced the death of relatives, parents, and friends. In this context it again was difficult for me to try to maintain the balance between closeness and distance; in this case the humanness allowed me to get close, even if all the information was collected with the research in mind.

Methodologically speaking, my work during the interviews was similar to that presented by Rosenthal (2004), even if the stories I collected concentrated on a particular segment of life during an earthquake experience. According to Rosenthal, the analysis of the interview data, the so-called biographical case reconstruction of an interview, consists of the following steps:

- Analysis of the (objective) biographical data
- Text and thematic field analysis (structure of self-presentation; reconstruction of the life story; narrated life)
- Reconstruction of the life history (lived life as experienced)
- Microanalysis of individual text segments
- Contrasting comparison of life history (experienced life) and life story (narrated life)
- Development of types and contrastive comparison of several cases

I followed this plan but I changed it regarding the microanalysis and the comparison because it was not about only the singular life stories but about the three earthquakes as different events and contexts to be analyzed. I used the voices of victims of each earthquake as one main voice (multivoices) to tell and represent the earthquake experience. The final result overcomes fragmentary stories and their telling to provide readers with the homogeneity of "one long story" that is constituted from more than one voice.

Analyzing the original use of this approach for studying disaster resilience from a sociological perspective, I utilized and recognized the main methodological suggestions of Bertaux (1998) and Bichi (2000). In particular, I took into account the importance of creating an interview situation (Bertaux 1998) and the necessity of asking for clarifications during interviews at the right moment and with the right question.

I symbolically elaborated an autobiographical pact (Berger and Quinney 2005) with every interviewee to show respect to them and create trust and a social relationship out of our interviews, as well as to give the right consideration to their local knowledge.

I must confess that it was not possible to feel only "good" feelings of participation and solidarity. Sometimes, especially in Molise, I experienced many conflicting feelings, including frustration and impotence because of the difficulty of interviewing people and creating a relationship of trust and collaboration. Impotence was my main feeling during my time in L'Aquila and its surroundings because of the ghostly situation and context.

10.5 The Figure of the Researcher and Her Feelings

Another key issue within the methodological field was my personal positions and identity (Bertaux 1998) as a researcher. I was in my last year of my PhD course and it had been difficult to affirm for myself that "I am a researcher." My PhD thesis is the first research that I elaborated alone and used to prove my theoretical and methodological interests, so trying to consider myself as the figure of the researcher was not a simple act for me.

I observed in a reflexive, useful way that I was more able to use the identity of researcher within the context of semistructured interviews with the experts because I noted that this figure was more accepted by them than the figure of PhD student. Some experts also were interested in my research because the topic is quite similar to their jobs, and this fact facilitated my access in the institutional context and during their interviews.

However, what really surprised me was the impossibility of maintaining only one figure throughout the research process: sometimes I was known and recognized as a researcher, sometimes as a PhD student. The discriminating factor would have been the context – the cultural and the cognitive level of the participants in the research. As I said, in general I was a researcher for the experts and institutional personnel, and I preferred (and it was more useful) to be a PhD student when interacting with ordinary people and the population in general. Asking for an interview about deeply dramatic experiences such as earthquakes and, above all, asking this of people who had lost relatives, parents, and friends was not a simple thing to do.

I felt as though I was a sort of "thief of stories" or "thief of witness' voices," and it was not good feeling. During the interviews, mostly the first ones, I was frightened when people started to cry; I knew I was the reason for all that pain and I felt embarrassed and guilty. But when a person told me that it "felt good to tell this experience to another person" or someone said to me "thank you for listening to our stories," I understood that, even if there are always some exceptions to consider, many people affected by an earthquake – as well as other types of disasters – need to tell their experience to another. My strength was not in being a clinician. I was there, showing a real and deep interest in what they were telling me, and I was not interested in psychological or clinical mechanisms and dynamics, but instead, main reason for my being there was simply to listen. I think this made all the difference regarding the kind of information I was able to collect and the trust relationships that I established with the interviewees.

I am speaking also about the role and the use of scientific listening that is different from the simple listening of everyday life. During it I was interested in understanding the experiences lived by those people, and I kept in mind the guide for the dynamics I wanted to know and explore. The particular context of interviews created ambivalent feelings in myself toward different social groups such as ordinary people, institutional people, and technical and voluntary personnel; I had to be able to manage them all to safeguard the necessary level of participation and the possibility of analyzing the information collected.

This situation, even in an ethnographic context, was important for me and the relationships established with the people interviewed. As Hammersley and Atkinson (2007) note:

> Harm may also arise within ethnographic research from the nature of the field relations that are established. At the very least, being researched can create stress and provoke anxiety, especially if the researcher is believed to be evaluating one's work, one's life or oneself. . . . Ethnographers usually seek to build rapport and trust, so that these may be lessened or disappear in the course of the fieldwork. At the same time, there are dangers that can arise from successfully establishing close relations with people in the field, for the researcher, for them, or for both.

Another interesting feeling was my personal upset after some of the first touching interviews. I recorded and transcribed the interviews during and shortly after the interviews themselves to maintain the memory and their voices inside my mind, but then I was not able to read the same interviews again for some time after. I needed time to understand not only the social dynamics of my topic but also my own feelings and thoughts regarding the situation. I must learn to manage all these feelings in the best way possible to guarantee that these feelings will influence – although not too much – my next analysis.

It was a deep path of personal awareness, and the discussion of methodology also concerns this kind of trouble. Methodology means the way you try to arrive at a better knowledge about something of interest to you, and this requires a discussion about all your previous thinking and principles. In fact, trying to find a method and the adequate instruments to know more about what you are interested or what you thought it could be is the real challenge of the methodological aspects of any research project. The Molise earthquake and the life stories I collected there probably were the biggest examples of my methodological path and the importance of being aware of it and learning from it for future research projects.

10.6 Ethics in the Research Process

Ethical questions are always presented within research processes involving human and social science and, for this reason, people themselves. I had to think about different ethical aspects because of the diverse methodological instruments I decided to use for my research. However, I argue that the universal and basilar ethical principles of all research involving people are always present. These include:

- Respecting, protecting, and defending the participant of the research project
- Receiving informed consent for participation in the research
- Respecting the privacy of people and their anonymity when necessary or required. The issue of privacy is very important, especially when collecting people's life stories in their homes, and, in a different way, for all the other participants in research, in this case both experts as well as civil protection volunteers
- Telling the participants the real aim of the research and, if appropriate, also the research project, in the clearest way possible
- Respecting others' time. In this research this was true for ordinary people but above all for the experts who did not have as much time to dedicate to my research
- Recognizing other contributions about one's topic by international authors. My personal experience of contact with international academics and experts on disaster resilience confirms this important principle
- Not distorting or inventing data, information, or the findings of the research

I wanted to respect all these principles in my research because I deeply believe in the utility of research if done with the respect for the all participants and their personal and social features. Especially when collecting the people's life stories setting and interviewing the experts, I had to guarantee anonymity and respect their sorrow and pain and their position and reactions regarding the earthquake itself and not allow myself to ask useless polemical questions.

Appendix A

Outline of Interview with the Experts in the Italian Civil Protection System

Introduction to the Voluntary Issue

1. Who is the civil protection volunteer, for you?

Part 1: Voluntary Service in the Civil Protection Area

2. Can you define the typical person who becomes a civil protection volunteer?
3. What are, according to you, the differences between civil protection voluntary service and volunteer service in another area?

   (Motivations to become volunteers, attitudes and perceptions of their role)

4. According to you, what are the main motivations for becoming a civil protection volunteer? (for example, altruism, solidarity, social prestige, desire to participate, new knowledge/competencies)
5. Which roles did you assume (e.g., attitudes such as solidarity, collaboration, altruism, pro-sociality, and trust) within the activities of civil protection voluntary service?
6. Are there any peculiarities and/or differences when participating in civil protection volunteer services between different regions of Italy and, more specifically, between Umbria, Marche, Molise, and Abruzzo?

(There have been or there are differences or particular characteristics among diverse regions while participating in civil protection voluntary services, for example, regarding motivations, maintenance, or commitment.)

B. Lucini, *Disaster Resilience from a Sociological Perspective*, Humanitarian Solutions in the 21st Century, DOI 10.1007/978-3-319-04738-6,

Part 2: Relationship Between Volunteers and the Civil Protection Association

7. According to you, which characteristics mark the interactions between volunteers and your own association with particular reference to the earthquakes in Umbria and Marche (1997), Molise, (2002), and Abruzzo (2009)?

(For example, were collaborative interactions or conflicts established? Was the association based on a hierarchical model or sharing tasks, recognition and legitimation of specific roles?)

8. How, do you believe, did the volunteers committed to the same group interact during the earthquakes in Umbria and Marche (1997), Molise, (2002) and Abruzzo (2009)?

(For example, volunteers demonstrated behavior and attitudes of availability and collaboration for teamwork, a specific single role was recognized, or there was conflict and limited availability for teamwork—as the major feature of this type of interaction.)

9. Which roles did you assume, according to you (e.g., attitudes such as solidarity, collaboration, and trust among volunteers committed to the same group) during the earthquakes in Umbria and Marche (1997), Molise (2002) and Abruzzo (2009)?

(How did the presence or absence of these attitudes orient the relationships between volunteers during the different phases of the emergency for these critical events?)

Part 3: Relationship Between Civil Protection Volunteers and the Population Affected by Critical Events

10. Who, for the population, is the civil protection volunteer?

(The volunteer is considered by the population as a helper, a useful, important person, or as a stranger, intrusive within the dynamics that existed before the critical event.)

11. Which kind of relationships were there between the volunteers and the population during the earthquakes in Umbria and Marche (1997), Molise (2002), and Abruzzo (2009)?

(Between the volunteers and the population, during the management phases of the critical event, was it possible to recognize solidarity and helpful relationships, conflicts and tension, or a mix of all of these, perhaps connected with the emergency management and its phases?)

Part 4: Conclusion

12. Which type of resources does the civil protection volunteer represent?
13. How have the social relationships that generally characterize volunteers changed over the years (between and within groups of volunteers and the population) and in particular referring to the earthquakes in Umbria and Marche (1997), Molise (2002) and Abruzzo (2009)?

(Has there been a change within voluntary relationships in terms of solidarity, collaboration, conflict, and tension referring to the considered critical events?)

Appendix B

Online Questionnaire

Introduction

This questionnaire has been developed for all civil protection volunteers who came from all regions of Italy during the Umbria and Marche (1997), Molise (2002) and Abruzzo (2009) earthquakes.

The aim of this research is to understand the features of civil protection voluntary activities, and the relationships established between volunteers and the population affected by earthquakes, to comprehend the way in which a community stricken by such a disaster copes with and faces the issues during the initial impact and during the reconstruction phase.

To do this, we kindly ask for your availability to fill out the present online questionnaire following the criteria you will find there.

Thank you for your collaboration.

Online Questionnaire

Part1: Personal and Social Data

1. How old are you?
2. Sex?
   - M
   - F
3. Region of permanent address
4. Which is your educational level?

B. Lucini, *Disaster Resilience from a Sociological Perspective*, Humanitarian Solutions in the 21st Century, DOI 10.1007/978-3-319-04738-6,

- Primary school
- Secondary school
- High school (technical or other)
- Bachelor's degree
- Master's degree

Part 2: Civil Protection Voluntary Service

5. When did you begin to be a civil protection volunteer?
6. What motives have determined your choice to be a civil protection volunteer?

   More than one answer is possible.

   - Offering help
   - Listening to people during their moment of need
   - Availability of free time
   - Desire to experience and live within a group
   - Generosity
   - A sense of civic responsibility
   - Donate something of yourself
   - Possibility of enhancing yourself
   - Possibility of enhancing your professionalism
   - Be a point of reference to those who are in difficulty
   - Having grown up in a family where voluntary service is considered an important activity
   - Curiosity
   - Personal expectations
   - To affirm religious values or be approved by your religion
   - Other (please specify)

7. To which kind of voluntary service organization do you belong?

   - Association
   - Local group (municipality)
   - Interlocal group

8. Who is the decision maker within your organization of voluntary service?

   - The president of the voluntary association or the coordinator of the voluntary group along with the volunteers
   - The president of the voluntary association or the coordinator of the voluntary group
   - Meeting of all volunteers or their delegation after group discussions
   - The volunteers

9. How do you define your relationship with your own group of volunteers (peers) in a time of no emergency (e.g., normal activities of voluntary service, meeting, bringing up to date, training)?

   More than one answer is possible.

   - Collaborative
   - Trusting
   - Reciprocal help
   - Friendly
   - Conflicting
   - Competitive
   - Rivalry

10. How do you define your relationship with your own group of volunteers (peers) in a time of emergency? More than one answer is possible.

    - Collaborative
    - Trusting
    - Reciprocal help
    - Friendly
    - Conflicting
    - Competitive
    - Rivalry

11. Do you agree with the norms of your own voluntary service organization?

    - Strongly agree
    - Somewhat agree
    - Somewhat disagree
    - Strongly disagree
    - Neutral

12. In your opinion, which role does a civil protection volunteer primarily take?

    - Training citizens
    - Assisting the population affected by the critical event
    - Answering the primary needs of the population
    - Disseminating preventive practices and behaviour
    - Technical and logistical management of relief aid
    - Emotional management of the population
    - Other (please specify)

13. How do you feel about this sentence: "The first civil protection volunteer is the citizen herself/himself"?

    - Strongly agree
    - Somewhat agree
    - Somewhat disagree
    - Strongly disagree
    - Neutral

Part 3: Three Earthquake Experiences: Umbria and Marche in 1997, Molise in 2002, Abruzzo in 2009

14. In which of these three earthquakes did you participate as civil protection volunteer?

    More than one answer is possible.

    - Umbria and Marche 1997
    - Molise 2002
    - Abruzzo 2009

15. How long did you stay in the Umbria and Marche earthquake area?

    - Less than 7 days
    - 1 Week
    - 2 Weeks
    - Nearly 1 month
    - Up to 3 months
    - Up to 6 months
    - More than 6 months

16. How long did you stay in the Molise earthquake area?

    - Less than 7 days
    - 1 Week
    - 2 Weeks
    - Nearly 1 month
    - Up to 3 months
    - Up to 6 months
    - More than 6 months

17. How long did you stay in the Abruzzo earthquake area?

    - Less than 7 days
    - 1 Week
    - 2 Weeks
    - Nearly 1 month
    - Up to 3 months
    - Up to 6 months
    - More than 6 months

18. What kind of relationship did you establish with the population affected by the Umbria and Marche earthquake?

    - Helpful
    - Reciprocal collaboration
    - Emotional closeness
    - Problematic
    - Distant
    - Conflicting

19. What kind of relationship did you establish with the population affected by the Molise earthquake?
    - Help
    - Reciprocal collaboration
    - Emotional closeness
    - Problematic
    - Distant
    - Conflicting
20. Which kind of relationship did you establish with the population affected by the Abruzzo earthquake?
    - Helpful
    - Reciprocal collaboration
    - Emotional closeness
    - Problematic
    - Distant
    - Conflicting
21. Considering the Umbria and Marche earthquake, did the population affected by it demonstrate they had resources that were useful for an active and participative response to the emergency and available before the earthquake itself?
    - Yes, emotional
    - Yes, organizational
    - Yes, economic
    - Yes, social networks and friendships for helping
    - No
22. Considering the Molise earthquake, did the population affected by it demonstrate they had resources that were useful for an active and participative response to the emergency and available before the earthquake itself?
    - Yes, emotional
    - Yes, organizational
    - Yes, economic
    - Yes, social networks and friendships for helping
    - No
23. Considering the Molise earthquake, did the population affected by it demonstrate they had resources that were useful for an active and participative response to the emergency and available before the earthquake itself?
    - Yes, emotional
    - Yes, organizational
    - Yes, economic
    - Yes, social networks and friendships for helping
    - No

24. In what way do you think the population affected by an earthquake consider a volunteer?

    More than one answer is possible.

    - A helper during a time of need
    - A friend
    - A stranger
    - A person who organizes and manages useful services and activities

25. Did you have a continuing relationship with the population affected by the earthquakes?

    - Yes, for a short time after the emergency (12 months later)
    - Yes, with systematic contacts
    - Yes, with occasional contacts (birthdays, marriages, etc.)
    - No

26. How do you judge the following statements?

    - There is a lot of spontaneity and a rush of emotional enthusiasm for the response to the emergency.
    - Strongly agree
    - Somewhat agree
    - Somewhat disagree
    - Strongly disagree
    - Neutral
    - Professionalism and training has increased for volunteers who are involved in an emergency management.
    - Strongly agree
    - Somewhat agree
    - Somewhat disagree
    - Strongly disagree
    - Neutral
    - The organization of the emergency response has become more structured.
    - Strongly agree
    - Somewhat agree
    - Somewhat disagree
    - Strongly disagree
    - Neutral
    - The help given has changed: it is not only technical and operative but also listens to and supports the population affected by the disaster.
    - Strongly agree
    - Somewhat agree
    - Somewhat disagree
    - Strongly disagree
    - Neutral

- There is more agreement with the common rules during the emergency response.
- Strongly agree
- Somewhat agree
- Somewhat disagree
- Strongly disagree
- Neutral

Part 4: Conclusion

27. Do you consider training important in helping relationships with the population affected by disasters?

    - Yes
    - No

28. How do you judge your civil protection voluntary experience?

    - Very positive
    - Positive
    - Negative
    - Very negative

Appendix C

First Input for the Storytelling

Would you please tell me your experience of the earthquakes, starting with the description of your life and its organization (family, job, hobby, friends, etc.) 1 year before the earthquake itself?

1. Time before earthquake
   - 1.1. Family: previous experience of earthquakes
   - 1.2. Job
   - 1.3. Social relationships (social networks, community)
   - 1.4. Hobbies, interests
   - 1.5. Perception and memory of known places, spaces, house/home
   - 1.6. Existence of previous contacts with civil protection volunteers or knowledge of the civil protection system
2. The impact of the earthquake
   - 2.1. The first response to the emergency: immediate actions and behaviors
   - 2.2. The first help received: from whom, what was it and its duration
   - 2.3. The first help offered: to whom, what was it and its duration
   - 2.4. Perception and memory linked to space and time of the critical event
   - 2.5. Past and present social relationships as a resource to the emergency response
3. The immediate response to the emergency
   - 3.1. The first contact with a civil protection volunteer: how, when, where
   - 3.2. The figure of the civil protection volunteer during the first phases of emergency response: description and characteristics of the established relationship
   - 3.3. Past and present interpersonal and social relationships and their changes

B. Lucini, *Disaster Resilience from a Sociological Perspective*, Humanitarian Solutions in the 21st Century, DOI 10.1007/978-3-319-04738-6,

4. After impact

    4.1. New habitation within the civil protection area (mobility, organization, legitimacy, social and institutional, recognition): established relationship with the civil protection volunteer, space perception (institutional and not), typology and characteristics, new experienced identity
    4.2. Community perception and living together in the habitation prepared by civil protection: perception and experience of attitudes as cohesion, collaboration, conflict, social distance during the time together
    4.3. Old and new interpersonal and social relationships: changes and characteristics
    4.4. Images and roles of civil protection volunteers during this phase

5. Reconstruction

    5.1. New location and habitation
    5.2. Resources used for the reconstruction: typology, characteristics, and availability
    5.3. Provided and received help: to/from whom, what it was, its duration (perception of help)
    5.4. Image and role of civil protection volunteers during this phase

6. Reconstruction/mitigation

    6.1. New organization of own life and its changes
    6.2. Social relationships and their changes
    6.3. Experience for the future: training

References

Abel, N., & Langston, A. (2001). *Evolution of a social-ecological system: Adaptation and resilience in the New South Wales Rangelands 1850 to 2020*. Retrieved from http://www.cse.csiro.au/research/nswrangelands/pubs/popular_articles/Draft_Paper.pdf.

Abesamis, N. P. et al. (2006). *Social resilience: A literature review on building resilience into human marine communities in and around MPA networks*. MPA Networks Learning Partnership.

Abramowitz, S. (2005). The poor have become rich and the rich have become poor: Collective trauma in the Guinean Languette. *Social Science and Medicine, 61*, 2106–2118.

Adam, B., et al. (2000). *Risk society and beyond. Critical issues for social theory*. London: Sage.

Adger, N. W. (2000). Social and ecological resilience: Are they related? *Progress in Human Geography, 24*, 3.

Adger, W. N. (2003). Social capital, collective action and adaptation to climate change. *Economic Geography, 79*, 387–404.

Adger, W. N., Hughes, T., Folke, C., Carpenter, S. R., & Rockström, J. (2005). Social-ecological resilience to coastal disasters. *Science, 309*, 1036–1039.

Aguirre, B. E. (2006). *On the concept of resilience* (Vol. Preliminary Paper #356). University of Delaware Disaster Research Center.

Ahmed, R., Seedat, M., van Niekerk, A., & Bulbulia, S. (2004). Discerning community resilience in disadvantaged communities in the context of violence and injury prevention. *South African Journal of Psychology, 34*, 386–408.

Alexander, D. (1993). *Natural disasters*. London/Dordrecht and Boston: University College London Press/Kluwer Academic.

Alexander, D. (2000). *Confronting catastrophe: New perspectives on natural disasters*. Harpenden/New York, NY: Terra Publishing/Oxford University Press.

Alexander, D. (2002). From civil defence to civil protection – And back again. *Disaster Prevention and Management, 11*, 209–213.

Allenby, B., & Fink, J. (2005). Toward inherently secure and resilient societies. *Science, 309*, 1034–1036.

Almond A. G., Flanagan S. C., & Mundt R. J. (Eds.) (1973). *Crisis, choice, and change:Historical studies of political development*. Boston: Little, Brown and Company.

Anderies, J. M., Janssen, M. A., & Ostrom, E. (2004). A framework to analyze the robustness of social-ecological systems from an institutional perspective. *Ecology and Society, 9*, 18. Retrieved from http://www.ecologandsociety.org/vol9/iss1/art18.

Antonovsky, A., & Sourani, T. (1988). Family sense of coherence and family adaptation. *Journal of Marriage and the Family, 50*, 79–92.

B. Lucini, *Disaster Resilience from a Sociological Perspective*, Humanitarian Solutions in the 21st Century, DOI 10.1007/978-3-319-04738-6,

Bachrach, K. M., & Zautra, A. J. (1985). Coping with a community stressor: The threat of a hazardous waste facility. *Journal of Health and Social Behavior, 26*, 127–141.

Bankoff, G. (2004). The historical geography of disaster: "Vulnerability" and "local knowledge" in western discourse. In G. Bankoff, G. Frerks, & D. Hilhorst (Eds.), *Mapping vulnerability. Disasters development and people*. London: Earthscan Publications.

Barton, A. H. (1963). *Social organization under stress: A sociological review of disaster studies*. Washington, DC: National Academy of Sciences, National Research Council.

Bateson, M. C. (1994). *Peripheral visions*. New York, NY: HarperCollins.

Bauman, Z. (1999). *La società dell'incertezza*. Bologna: Il Mulino.

Bauman, Z. (2001). *Voglia di comunità*. Bari: Laterza.

Bauman, Z. (2006a). *Vita liquida*. Bari: Laterza.

Bauman, Z. (2006b). *Liquid fear*. Cambridge: Polity Press.

Beato, F. (1998). *Rischio e mutamento ambientale globale: percorsi di sociologia dell'ambiente*. Milano: F. Angeli.

Beck, U. (1986). *Risikogesellschaft: Auf den Weg in eine andere Moderne*. Frankfurt: Suhrkamp.

Beck, U. (1992). From industrial society to the risk society: Questions of survival, social structure and ecological enlightenment. *Theory, Culture & Society, 9*, 97–123.

Beck, U. (2001). *La società globale del rischio*. Trieste: Asterios.

Beck, U. (2003). *Un mondo a rischio*. Torino: Einaudi.

Berger, P. L., & Luckmann, T. (1966). *The social construction of reality*. New York, NY: Garden City.

Berger, J., & Quinney, R. (2005). *Storytelling sociology: Narrative as social inquiry*. Boulder, CO: Linne Rienner Publishers.

Berkes, F., Folke, C., & Gadgil, M. (1995). Traditional knowledge, biodiversity, resilience, and sustainability. In C. A. Perrings, K.-G. Mäler, C. Folke, C. S. Holling, & B. O. Jansson (Eds.), *Biodiversity conservation*. Dordrecht: Kluwer Academic.

Bertaux, D. (1998). *Récits de vie*. Paris: Nathan.

Bertaux, D. (1999). Les effets du témoignage. In R. Dulong & P. Gruson (Eds.), *L'Expérience du déni*. Paris: Éditions de la Maison des Sciences de l'Homme.

Bertaux. D. (1976). *Histoires de vie – ou récits de pratiques? Méthodologie de l'approche biographique en sociologie*. Rapport au CORDES.

Bichi, R. (2000). *La società raccontata. Metodi biografici e vite complesse*. Milano: F. Angeli.

Bichi, R. (2002). *L'intervista biografica*. Milano: Vita e Pensiero.

Bichi, R. (2007). The life story as interview: Researching the trajectories of out of family children in Bosnia and Herzegovina. *Cogniţie, Creier, Comportament/Cognition, Brain, Behavior, Romanian Association for Cognitive Science, XI*.

Bichi, R. (2007b). *La conduzione delle interviste nella ricerca sociale*. Roma: Carocci.

Birkmann, J. (2006). *Measuring vulnerability to natural hazards: Toward disaster resilient societies*. Tokyo, New York, Paris: United Nations University Press.

Blaikie, P., et al. (1994). *At risk: Natural hazards, people's vulnerability, and disasters* (1st ed.). London: Routledge.

Blumenfield, M., & Ursano, R. J. (2008). *Intervention and resilience after mass trauma*. Cambridge: Cambridge University Press.

Bodin, P., & Wiman, B. (2004). Resilience and other stability concepts in ecology: Notes on their origin, validity, and usefulness. *ESS Bulletin, 2*, 33–43.

Bogardi, J. J. (2006). *Resilience building: From knowledge to action. Introduction to UNU-EHS*. Presented to the Summer Academy of UNU: EHS, June. Retrieved from http://www.ehs.unu.edu/file.php?id=184.

Bogardi, J., & Birkmann, J. (2004). Vulnerability assessment: The first step towards sustainable risk reduction. In D. Malzahn & T. Plapp (Eds.), *Disaster and society – From hazard assessment to risk reduction*. Berlin: Logos Verlag Berlin.

Bohle, H. G. (2001). *Vulnerability and criticality: Perspectives from social geography*. IHDP Update 2/2001. Newsletter of the International Human Dimensions Programme on Global Environmental Change.

Bohle, H.-G. (2007). Leben mit Risiko: Resilience als neues Paradigma für die Risikowelten von morgen. In C. Felgentreff & T. Glade (Eds.), *Naturrisiken und Sozialkatastrophen*. Heidelberg: Elsevier/Spektrum Akademischer Verlag).

Boin, A., & Hart, P. (2006). The crisis approach. In H. Rodriguez, E. Quarantelli, & R. R. Dynes (Eds.), *Handbook of disaster research*. NY: Springer.

Bollin, C. (2003). *Community-based disaster risk management approach*. Eschborn: ETZ. Division 4200 Governance and Democracy.

Bonanno, G. A. (2004). Loss, trauma, and human resilience: Have we underestimated the human capacity to thrive after extremely aversive events? *American Psychologist, 59*, 20–28.

Bonanno, G. A., et al. (2002). Resilience to loss and chronic grief: A prospective study from pre-loss to 18-months postloss. *Journal of Personality and Social Psychology, 83*, 1150–1164.

Bonanno, G. A., et al. (2010). Weighing the costs of disaster: consequences, risks, and resilience in individuals, families, and communities. *Psychological Science in the Public Interest, 11*, 1–49.

Bourdieu, P. (1983/1986). The forms of capital. In J. G. Richardson (Ed.), *Handbook of theory and research in the sociology of education*. Westport, CT: Greenwood Press.

Brand, F. S., & Jax, K. (2007). Focusing the meaning(s) of resilience: Resilience as a descriptive concept and a boundary object. *Ecology and Society, 12,* 23. Retrieved from http://www.ecologyandsociety.org/vol12/iss1/art23/.

Bravo, M., Rubio-Stipec, M., Canino, G. J., Woodbury, M. A., & Ribera, J. C. (1990). The psychological sequelae of disaster stress prospectively and retrospectively evaluated. *American Journal of Community Psychology, 18*, 661–680.

Brenson-Lazan, G. (2003). *Group and social resilience building*. Retrieved from www.communityatwork.com/resilience/RESILIENCIAENG.pdf.

Breton, M. (2001). Neighborhood resiliency. *Journal of Community Practice, 19*, 21–36.

Brock, W. A., Mäler, K.-G., & Perrings, C. (2002). Resilience and sustainability: The economic analysis of nonlinear systems. In L. H. Gunderson & C. S. Holling (Eds.), *Panarchy: Understanding transformations in systems of humans and nature*. Washington, DC: Island Press.

Bronfenbrenner, U. (1996). Modèle "Processus-Personne-COntexte-Temps". In *Le modèle ecologique dans l'ètude du développement de l'enfant*. Quèbec: Presses Universitaires.

Brown, D., & Kulig, J. (1996/1997). The concept of resiliency: Theoretical lessons from community. *Research, Health and Canadian Society, 4*, 29–52.

Bruneau, M., et al. (2003). A framework to quantitatively assess and enhance the seismic resilience of communities. *Earthquake Spectra, 19*, 733–752.

Butler, L., Morland, L., & Leskin, G. (2007). Psychological resilience in the face of terrorism. In B. Bongar, L. Brown, L. Beutler, J. Breckenridge, & P. Zimbardo (Eds.), *Psychology of terrorism* (pp. 400–417). New York, NY: Oxford University Press.

Callero, P. L., Howard, J. A., & Piliavin, J. A. (1987). Helping behavior as a role behavior: Disclosing social structure and history on the analysis of prosocial action. *Social Psychology Quarterly, 50*, 247–256.

Cannon, T., Twigg, J., & Rowell, J. (2003). *Social vulnerability. Sustainable livelihoods and disasters*. Report to DFID Conflict and Humanitarian Assistance Department (CHAD) and Sustainable Livelihoods Support Office. Retrieved from http://www.abuhrc.org/Pages/index.aspxdisaster_studies/projects/soc_vuln_sust_live.pdf.

Carpenter, S., et al. (2001). From metaphor to measurement: Resilience of what to what? *Ecosystems, 4*, 765–781.

Carr, L. J. (1932). Disaster and the sequence pattern concept of social change. *American Journal of Sociology, 38*, 207–218.

Castelli, C. (2011). *Resilienza e creatività*. Milano: Franco Angeli.

Cattarinussi, B., & Pelanda C. (Eds.) (1981). *Disastro e azione umana Introduzione multidisciplinare allo studio del comportamento sociale in ambienti estremi.* Milano: Franco Angeli.

Center for Community Enterprise (2000). Retrieved from http://www.cedworks.com/files/pdf/free/MW100410.pdf.

Chacòn, F. et al. (2006). The three stage model of volunteers' duration. In *Comunicazione al 2006 Biennial Meeting of the Society Psychological Study of Social Issues, Long Beach, CA, June 23–25.*

Chambers, R., & Conway, G. R. (1992). *Sustainable rural livelihoods: Practical concepts for the 21st century* (Discussion Paper 296). Brighton: Institute of Development Studies.

Chenoweth, L., & Stehlik, D. (2001). Building resilient communities: Social work practice and rural Queensland. *Australian Social Work, 54*(2), 47–54.

Choi et al. (2010). *How do groups react to unexpected threats? Crisis management in organizational teams.* Retrieved from http://findarticles.com/p/articles/mi_7398/is_6_38/ai_n55089796/.

Cicchetti, D. (1996). Developmental theory: Lessons from the study of risk and psychopathology. In S. Matthysse, D. L. Levy, J. Kagan, & F. M. Benes (Eds.), *Psychopathology: The evolving science of mental disorder* (pp. 253–284). New York, NY: Cambridge University Press.

Cicchetti, D., & Rogosch, F. A. (1997). The role of self-organization in the promotion of resilience in maltreated children. *Development and Psychopathology, 9*, 797–815.

Clarke, R. (1989). *Knowledge-based expert systems: Risk factors and potentially profitable application areas*. Retrieved from www.rogerclarke.com/SOS/KBTE.html.

Clausen, L. (1992). Social differentiation and the long term origin of disasters. *Natural Hazards, 6*, 181–190.

Clausen, L. (1994). *Krasser sozialer Wandel.* Opladen; Leske+Budrich (Kieler Beiträge zur Politik und Sozialwissenschaft Bd. 8).

Clausen, L., & Dombrowsky, W. R. (1983). *Einghurung in die Soziologieder katastrophen*. Bonn: Osang Verlag.

Clausen, L., Geenen, E. M., & Macamo, E. (2003). *Entsetzliche soziale Prozesse Theorie und Empirie der Katastrophen. Konflikte, Krisen und Katastrophen.* LIT-Verlag (sozialer und kultureller Sicht Bd. 1).

Clausen, L., & Jager, M. (1975). Zur Sociologischen Katastrophenanalze. *Zivilverterdigung, 4*, 20–24.

Clausen, L., et al. (1978). New aspects of the sociology of disaster: A theoretical note. *Mass Emergencies, 3*, 61–65.

Clauss-Ehlers, C. S., & Lopez Levy, L. (2002). Violence and community, terms in conflict: An ecological approach to resilience. *Journal of Social Distress and the Homeless, 11*(4), 265–278.

Clavandier, G. (2004). *La mort collective: pour une sociologie des catastrophes*. Paris: CNRS.

Cohen, S. (1992). Stress, social support, and disorder. In H. Veiel & U. Baumann (Eds.), *The meaning and measurement of social support*. New York, NY: Hemisphere.

Cohler, B. J., Stott, F. M., & Musicj, J. S. (1995). Adversity, vulnerability, and resilience: Cultural and developmental perspectives. In D. Cicchetti & D. J. Cohen (Eds.), *Risk, disorder, and adaptation* (Developmental psychopathology: Vol. 2, pp. 753–800). New York, NY: Wiley.

Coles, E., & Buckle, P. (2004). Developing community resilience as a foundation for effective disaster recovery. *Australian Journal of Emergency Management, 19*, 6–15.

Comfort, L. (1999). *Shared risk: Complex systems in seismic response*. New York, NY: Pergamon.

Corbetta, P. (1999). *Metodologia e tecniche della ricerca sociale*. Bologna: il Mulino.

Cutter, S. (2003). The science of vulnerability and the vulnerability of science. *Annals of the Association of American Geographers, 93*(1), 1–12.

Cutter, S. L., Barnes, L., Berry, M., Burton, C., Evans, E., Tate, E., & Webb, J. (2008). A place-based model for understanding community resilience to natural disasters. *Global Environmental Change, 18*, 598–606.

Cutter, S. L., Boruff, B. J., & Shirley, W. L. (2003). Social vulnerability to environmental hazards. *Social Science Quarterly, 84*, 242–261.

Cutter, S., Burton, C., & Emrich, C. (2010). Disaster resilience indicators for benchmarking baseline conditions. *Journal of Homeland Security and Emergency Management, 7*, 51.

Cyrulnik, B., & Malaguti E. (Eds.) (2005). *Costruire la resilienza. La riorganizzazione positiva della vita e la creazione di legami positivi.* Trento: Erickson.

Davis, M. (2005). Becoming (and remaining) a community volunteer: Does personality matter? In A. M. Omoto (Ed.), *Process of community change and social action. The Claremont symposium on applied social psychology*. Mahwah, NJ: Lawrence Erlbaum Associates.

De Marchi, B., et al. (2001). *Il rischio ambientale*. Bologna: Il Mulino.
Denney, D. (2005). *Risk society*. Thousand Oaks, CA: Sage.
Di Sopra, L., & Pelanda C. (Eds.) (1984). *Teoria della vulnerabilità*. Milano: F. Angeli.
Dietz, T., & Rycroft, R. W. (1987). *The risk professionals*. New York, NY: Russell Sage.
Dietz, T., Stern, P. C., & Rycroft, R. W. (1989). Definitions of conflicts and the legitimation of resources: The case of environmental risk. *Sociological Forum, 4*, 47–70.
Subcommittee on Disaster Reduction (2005). *Grand challenges for disaster reduction*. Washington, DC: National Science & Technology Council, Committee on Environment and Natural Resources.
Dombrowsky, W. R. (1981). *Another step toward a social theory of disaster* (Preliminary Paper #70). University of Delaware Disaster Research Centre.
Dombrowsky, W. R. (1989). *Katastrophe und katastrophenschutz Eine soziologische Analyse*. Wiesbaden: Dt. Universitätsverlag.
Donati, P. (2007a). Building a relational theory of society: A sociological journey. In M. Deflem (Ed.), *Sociologists in a global age. Biographical perspectives* (pp. 159–174). Aldershot: Ashgate.
Donati, P. (2007b). Capitale sociale, reti associazionali e beni relazionali. *Impresa Sociale, 76*, 168–191.
Donati, P. (2007c). Introduzione: perché la sociologia relazionale? *Nuova Civiltà delle Macchine, XXV*, 7–26.
Douglas, M. (1991). *Come percepiamo il pericolo: antropologia del rischio*. Milano: Feltrinelli.
Douglas, M. (1996). *Rischio e colpa*. Bologna: Il Mulino.
Douglas, M., & Wildavsky, A. (1982). *Risk and culture*. Berkeley, CA: University of California Press.
Downing, T. E. et al. (2006). *Integrating social vulnerability into water management* (SEI Working Paper and Newater Working Paper No. 4). Oxford: Stockholm Environment Institute.
Drabek, T. E. (2010). *The human side of disaster*. Boca Raton, FL: Taylor and Francis Group.
Durkheim, E. (1893: 1897). *La Division du travail social*. Paris: Presses Universitaires de France.
Dynes, R. (1994). *Situational altruism: Toward an explanation of pathologies in disaster assistance* (Preliminary Paper #201). University of Delaware Disaster Research Centre.
Dynes, R. (2002). *The importance of social capital in disaster response* (Preliminary Paper #327). University of Delaware Disaster Research Centre.
Dynes, R. R., et al. (1987). *Sociology of disaster*. Milano: F. Angeli.
Egeland, B., Carlson, E., & Sroufe, L. A. (1993). Resilience as process. *Development and Psychopathology, 5*, 517–528.
Eisner, R. (2009). *Disaster resilient organizations*. Bay Area Preparedness Initiative. Retrieved from http://www.resilientus.org/wp-content/uploads/2013/03/Richard_Eisner_1248897598.pdf.
Elias, N. (1986). *Saggio sul tempo*. Bologna: Il Mulino.
emBRACE (2012). Systematization of different concepts, quality criteria, and indicators. Working Paper. Work Package 1, Deliverable 1.2.
Enarson, E. (2006). *Women and girls last? Averting the second post-katrina disaster.* Social Science Research Council. Retrieved from http://understandingkatrina.ssrc.org/Enarson.
Enarson, E. (2007). Identifying and addressing social vulnerabilities. In *Emergency management: Principles and practice for local government* (2nd ed.). Retrieved from www.training.fema.gov.
Enarson, E. (2010). A gendered human rights approach to rebuilding after disaster. In A. Awatona (Ed.), *Rebuilding sustainable communities for children and their families after disaster: A global survey*. Newcastle: Cambridge Scholars Publishing.
Enarson, E., & Dhar Chakrabarti, P. G. (2010). *Women, gender and disaster. Global issues and initiatives*. New Delhi: Sage.
Evers, A., & Nowotny, H. (1987). *Über den Umgang mit Unsicherheit. Die Entdeckung der Gestaltbarkeit von Gesellschaft*. Frankfurt a. M.: Suhrkamp.
Falck, H. (1994). *La prospettiva dell'appartenenza nel servizio sociale*. Milano: Vita e Pensiero.
Felgentreff, C., & Glade, T. (2008). *Naturrisiken und Sozialkatastrophen*. Berlin: Spektrum Akademischer Verlag Gmbh.

Fischer, H. W. (2003). The sociology of disaster: Definitions, research questions, & measurements. *International Journal of Mass Emergencies and Disasters, 1*, 91–107 (continuation of the discussion in a post-September 11 environment).
Fritz, C. E. (1961). Disasters. In R. K. Merton & R. A. Nisbet (Eds.), *Contemporary social problems*. New York, NY: Harcourt, Brace & World.
Gallopin, G. C. (2006). Linkages between vulnerability, resilience and adaptive capacity. *Global Environmental Change, 16*, 293–303.
Ganor, M., & Ben-Lavy, Y. (2003). Community resilience: Lessons derived from Gilo under Fire. *Journal of Jewish Communal Service, Winter/Spring*, 105–108.
Garbarino, J., et al. (1992). *Children in danger: Coping with the consequences of community violence*. San Francisco: Jossey-Bass.
Garmezy, N. (1985). Stress-resistant children: The search for protective factors. In J. E. Stevenson (Ed.), *Recent research in developmental psychopathology [Book supplement no. 4 to Journal of Child Psychology and Psychiatry]* (pp. 213–233). Oxford: Pergamon.
Garmezy, N. (1991). Resiliency and vulnerability to adverse developmental outcomes associated with poverty. *American Behavioral Scientist, 34*, 416–430.
Gergen, K. J. (1994). *Realities and relationships: Soundings in social construction*. Cambridge, MA: Harvard University Press.
Gilbert, C. (1995). Studying disaster: A review of the main conceptual tools. *International Journal of Mass Emergencies and Disasters, 13*, 231–240.
Ginige, K., Amaratunga, D., & Haigh, R. (2009). Mainstreaming gender in disaster reduction: Why and how? *Disaster Prevention and Management., 18*, 23–34.
Godbout, J. T. (1992). *Lo spirito del dono*. Torino: Bollati Boringhieri.
Godschalk, D. (2003). Urban hazard mitigation: Creating resilient cities. *Natural Hazards Review, 4*, 136–143.
Gordon, J. (1978). *Structures*. Harmondsworth: Penguin Books.
Guèno, J. P. (2002). Paroles d'étoiles: Mémorie d'enfants cachés 1939–1945. Librio Document, Paris.
Gunderson, L. H., & Folke, C. (2005). Resilience—Now more than ever (editorial). *Ecology and Society, 10*. Retrieved from http://www.ecologyandsociety.org/vol10/iss2/art22/.
Habermas, J. (1975). *Legitimation crisis*. Boston: Beacon Press.
Habermas, J. (1980). *Agire comunicativo e logica delle scienze sociali*. Bologna: Il Mulino (ed. tr 1967, 1981).
Halbwachs, M. (1987). *La Memoria collettiva*. Milano: Unicopli.
Hammerl, C., et al. (2009). *Naturkatastrophen Rezeption – Bewaeltigung – Verarbeitung*. Wien: StudienVerlag.
Hammersley, M., & Atkinson, P. (2007). *Ethnography: Principles in Practice*. Abingdon: Routledge.
Heijmans, A. (2001). *Vulnerability: A matter of perception*. Paper Given at International Work-Conference Vulnerability in Disaster Theory and Practice. Wageningen Disaster Studies 29/30 June 2001.
Herman, C. F. (Ed.). (1972). *International crises: Insights from behavioral research*. New York, NY: Free Press.
Hobfoll, S. E., Ennis, N., & Kay, J. (2000). Loss, resources, and resilience in close interpersonal relationships. In J. H. Harvey & E. D. Miller (Eds.), *Loss and trauma: General and close relationship perspectives* (pp. 267–285). Philadelphia, PA: Brunner-Routledge.
Hoffman, L. (1990). Constructing realities: An art of lenses. *Family Process, 29*, 1–12.
Holling, C. S. (1973). Resilience and stability of ecological systems. *Annual Review of Ecology and Systematics, 4*, 1–23. Retrieved from http://www.jstor.org/discover/10.2307/2096802?uid=3738296&uid=2134&uid=2&uid=70&uid=4&sid=21103764429807.
Holling, C. S., & Gunderson, L. H. (2002). Resilience and adaptive cycles. In L. H. Gunderson & C. S. Holling (Eds.), *Panarchy. Understanding transformations in human and natural systems*. Washington: Island Press.
Holling, C. S., Schindler, D. W., Walker, B. W., & Roughgarden, J. (1995). Biodiversity in the functioning of ecosystems: An ecological synthesis. In C. Perrings, K. G. Maler, C. Folke, C.

S. Holling, & B. O. Jansson (Eds.), *Biodiversity loss: Economic and ecological issues* (pp. 44–83). Cambridge: Cambridge University Press.
Izzo, A. (1991). *Storia del pensiero sociologico*. il Mulino, Bologna.
Jaeger, W. (1977). *Katastrophe und Gesellschaft Grundlegungen und Kritik von Modellen del Katastrophensoziologie*. Darmstadt, Neuwied: Luchterhand.
Japp, K. P. (1996). *Soziologische Risikotheorie. Funktionale Differenzierung, Politisierung und Reflexion*. Weinheim, München: Juventa Verlag.
Japp, K. P. (2000). *Risiko*. Bielefeld, Transcript.
Japp, K. P. (2003). Zur Soziologie der Katastrophe. In L. Clausen, E.M. Geenen.
Jasanoff, S. (1986). *Risk management and political culture*. New York, NY: Russell Sage Foundation.
Jüngermann, H., Kasperson, R. E., & Wiedemann, P. M. (Eds.). (1989). *Risk Communication. Proceedings of the International Workshop on Risk Communication, October 17–21, 1988, Jülich*. Jülich, FRG: Kernforschungsanlage Jülich.
Kaniasty, K. (2011). Parental crucibles: Families coping with disaster. In P. Buchwald, K. Moore, & T. Ringeisen (Eds.), *Stress and anxiety: Application to education and health* (pp. 83–93). Berlin: Logos Verlag.
Kaniasty, K. (2012). Predicting social psychological well-being following trauma: The role of postdisaster social support. *Trauma: Theory, Research, Practice, Policy, 4*, 22–33.
Kaniasty, K., & Norris, F. (1995). In search of altruistic community: patterns of social support mobilization following hurricane hugo. *American Journal of Community Psychology, 23*, 447–477.
Kaniasty, K., & Norris, F. (2004). Social support in the aftermath of disasters,catastrophes, and acts of terrorism: Altruistic, overwhelmed, uncertain, antagonistic, and patriotic communities. In R. J. Ursano, A. E. Norwood, & C. S. Fullerton (Eds.), *Bioterrorism: Psychological and public health interventions*. Cambridge: Cambridge University Press.
Kaplan, S., & Garrick, B. J. (1981). On the quantitative definition of risk. *Risk Analysis, 1*, 11–27.
Kasperson, R. E., & Kasperson, J. X. (1983). Determining the acceptability of risk: Ethical and policy issues. In J. T. Rogers & D. V. Bates (Eds.), *Assessment and perception of risk to human health, conference proceedings* (pp. 135–155). Ottawa: Royal Society of Canada.
Kasperson, R. E., et al. (1988). The social amplification of risk: A conceptual framework. *Risk Analysis, 8*(2), 177–187.
Kendra, J., & Wachtendorf, T. (2003). Elements of resilience after the World Trade Center disaster: Reconstituting New York City's emergency operations centre. *Disasters, 27*, 37–53.
Kieffer, C. (1984). Citizen empowerment: A developmental perspective. *Prevention in Human Services, 3*, 9–36.
Kimhi, S., & Shamai, M. (2004). Community resilience and the impact of stress: Adult response to Israel's withdrawal from Lebanon. *Journal of Community Psychology, 32*, 439–451.
Klein, R., Nicholls, R., & Thomalla, F. (2003). Resilience to natural hazards: How useful is this concept? *Environmental Hazards, 5*, 35–45.
Koetter, T. (2004). *Risks and opportunities of urbanisation and megacities*. Athens: Risk and Disaster Prevention and Management.
Kofinas, G. (2003). Resilience of human-rangifer systems: Frames off resilience help to inform studies of human dimensions of change and regional sustainability. *IHDP Update, 2*, 6–7.
Krimsky, S., & Golding, D. (1992). *Social theories of risk*. London: Praeger.
Kuhlicke, C. (2013). Resilience: A capacity and a myth: findings from an in-depth case study in disaster management research. *Natural Hazards, 67*, 61–76.
Lagadec, P. (1991). *La gestion des crises. Outils de reflexion lÐusage des decideurs*. Paris: McGraw Hill.
Lagadec, P. (1994). *Crisis management: Come affrontare e gestire emergenze e imprevisti*. Milano: F. Angeli.
Lash, S. (2000). Risk culture. In B. Adam et al. (Eds.), *The risk society and beyond*. London: Sage.
Layne, C. M., Warren, J. S., Watson, P. J., & Shalev, A. Y. (2007). Risk, vulnerabilities, resistance and resilience: Towards integrated conceptualization of posttraumatic adaptation. In M. J.

Friedman, T. M. Keane, & P. A. Watson (Eds.), *Handbook of PTSD, science and practice* (pp. 497–520). New York, NY: Guilford Press.
Lett, J. (1990). Emics and etics: Notes on the epistemology of anthropology. In T. N. Headland, K. L. Pike, & M. Harris (Eds.), *Emics and etics. The insider/outsider debate*. Newbury Park: Sage.
Levine, C. (2004). The concept of vulnerability in disaster research. *Journal of Traumatic Stress, 17*, 395–402.
Lichtenberg, J., & Maclean, D. (1991). The role of the media in risk communication. In R. Kasperson & P. Stallen (Eds.), *Communicating risks to the public: International perspectives*. Ixjndon: Kluwer Academic.
Lichtenstein, S., Slovic, P., Fischhoff, B., Layman, M., & Combs, B. (1978). Judged frequency of lethal events. *Journal of Experimental Psychology: Human Learning and Memory, 4*, 551–578.
Licursi, S. (2010). *Sociologia della solidarietà*. Roma: Carocci editore.
Lin, N. (2002). *Social capital: A theory of social structure and action*. London: Cambridge University Press.
Linz, J. J., & Stepan, A. (1978). *The breakdown of democratic regimes*. Baltimore and London: The Johns Hopkins University Press.
Liu, J., et al. (2007). Complexity of coupled human and natural systems. *Science, 317*, 1513–1516.
Lombardi, M. (1997a). *Rischio ambientale e comunicazione*. Milano: F. Angeli.
Lombardi, M. (1997b). Media studies. *International Journal of Mass Emergencies and Disasters, 15*, 103–116.
Lombardi, M. (2005). *Comunicare nell'emergenza*. Milano: Vita e Pensiero.
Longstaff, P. (2005). *Security, resilience, and communication in unpredictable environments such as terrorism, natural disasters, and complex technology*. Syracuse, New York: Author.
Lorenz, D. F. (2013). The diversity of resilience: Contributions from a social science perspective. *Natural Hazards, 67*, 7–24.
Low, S., & Airman, I. (1992). *Place attachment*. New York, NY: Plenum Press.
Lucini, B. (2013). Social capital and sociological resilience in megacities contexts. *International Journal of Disaster Resilience in the Built Environment, 4*, 58–71.
Luhmann, N. (1991). *Soziologie des Risikos*. Berlin: de Gruyter (trad. it. Sociologia del rischio, Bruno Mondadori, Milano1996).
Luhmann, N. (1993). *Risk: A sociological theory*. Berlin: De Gruyter.
Lupton, D. (1999). *Risk*. London: Routledge.
Lupton, D. (2002). *Il rischio: percezione, simboli, culture*. Bologna: Il Mulino.
Luthar, S. S., Cicchetti, D., & Becker, B. (2000). The construct of resilience: A critical evaluation and guidelines for future work. *Child Development, 71*, 543–562.
Macamo, Elísio (Ed.). *Entsetzliche soziale Prozesse Theorie und Empirie der Katastrophen. Konflikte, Krisen und Katastrophen* – in sozialer und kultureller Sicht Bd. 1. LIT-Verlag.
MacLean, D. (1986). Social values and the distribution of risk. In D. MacLean (Ed.), *Values at risk* (pp. 75–93). Totowa: Rowman and Allanheld.
Madden, R. (2010). *Being ethnographic. A guide to the theory and practice of ethnography*. London: Sage.
Malaguti, E. (2005). *Educarsi alla resilienza. Come affrontare crisi e difficoltà e migliorarsi*. Trento: Erickson.
Margalit, A. (1998). *La società decente*. Milano: Guerini e Associati (ed. or. 1996).
Marincioni, F. (2003). *La gestione delle calamità naturali. Stati Uniti e Italia due culture a confronto*. Retrieved from http://ispro.it/wiki/images/d/dc/PC_Italia_usa.pdf.
Marinelli, A. (1993). *La costruzione sociale del rischio*. Milano: F. Angeli.
Marta, E., & Pozzi, M. (2007). *Psicologia del volontariato*. Roma: Carocci editore.
Masten, A. S. (2001). Ordinary magic: Resilience processes in development. *American Psychologist, 56*, 227–238.
Masten, A. S., Best, K., & Garmezy, N. (1990). Resilience and development: Contributions from the study of children who overcome adversity. *Development and Psychopathology, 2*, 425–444.

Mathbor, G. M. (2007). Enhancement of community preparedness for natural disasters. *International Social Work, 50*(3), 357–369.

Mayunga, J. S. (2007). *Understanding and applying the concept of community disaster resilience: A capital based approach.* Draft Paper Prepared for the Summer Academy for Social Vulnerability and Resilience Building, Munich, Germany.

Mazur, A. (1981). *The dynamics of technical controversy*. Washington, DC: Communications Press.

McDaniels, T. (2009). *Building resilience in regional infrastructure systems*. Boulder CRRA Resilience Meeting. Retrieved from http://www.resilientus.org/wpcontent/uploads/2013/03/Tim_McDaniels_1248886249.pdf.

McEntire, D. A. (2001). Triggering agents, vulnerabilities and disaster reduction: Towards a holistic paradigm. *Disaster Prevention and Management, 10*, 189–196.

Mead, G. H. (1934). *Mind, self and society*. Chicago, IL: The University of Chicago Press.

Mead, G. H. (1966). *Mente, Sé e società. Dal punto di vista di uno psicologo comportamentista*. Firenze: Editrice Universitaria G. Barbera.

Merton, R. K. (1949). *Social theory and social structure*. New York, NY: Free Press.

Mileti, D. (1999). *Disasters by design: A reassessment of natural hazards in the United States*. Washington, DC: Joseph Henry Press.

Miller, L. M. (2007). Collective disaster responses to Katrina and Rita: Exploring therapeutic community, social capital and social control. *Southern Rural Sociology, 22*, 45–65.

Miller, D. S., & Rivera, J. D. (2008). *Hurricane Katrina and the redefinition of landscape*. Lanham, MD: Lexington Books.

Morin, E. (1968). Pour une sociologie de la crise. *Communications, 12*, 2–16.

Morin, E. (1976). Pour une crisiologie. *Communications, 25*, 149–163.

Moscovici, S. (1994). Les formes elementaires de l'altruisme. In S. Moscovici (Ed.), *Psychologie Sociale de la relation à autrui. Paris: Nathan tr. it. La relazione con l'altro, 1997*. Milano: Cortina.

Murphy, R. (2009). *The leadership of disaster*. Kingston, ON: McGill Queen's University Press.

Nathan, F. (2005). *Vulnerabilities to natural hazard: Case study on landslide risks in La Paz*. Paper for the World International Studies Conference (WISC) at Bilgi University, Istanbul, Turkey, 24–27 August.

Neal, D. M. (1997). Reconsidering the phases of disaster. *International Journal of Mass Emergencies and Disasters, 15*, 239–264.

Nettles, S. M., Mucherah, W., & Jones, D. S. (2000). Understanding resilience: The role of social resources. *Journal of Education for Students Placed at Risk, 5*, 47–60.

Nigris, D. (2003). *Standard e non-standard nella ricerca sociale. Riflessioni metodologiche*. Milano: Franco Angeli.

Nixon, E., & Jaswal, H. K. (2010). Focusing the meaning(s) of resilience: Resilience as a descriptive concept and a boundary object. *Ecology and Society, 12,* 23. Retrieved from http://www.ecologyandsociety.org/vol12/iss1/art23/.

Norris, F. H., & Kaniasty, K. (1996). Received and perceived social support in times of stress: A test of the social support deterioration deterrence model. *Journal of Personality and Social Psychology, 71*, 498–511.

Norris, F. H., Stevens, S. P., Pfefferbaum, B., Wyche, K. F., & Pfefferbaum, R. L. (2008). Community resilience as a metaphor, theory, set of capacities, and strategy for disaster readiness. *American Journal of Community Psychology, 41*, 127–150.

Norris, F. H., et al. (2009). Looking for resilience: Understanding the longitudinal trajectories of responses to stress. *Social Science and Medicine, 68*, 2190–2198.

O'Riodan, T., Marrys, C., & Langford, I. (1997). Images of science underlying public perceptions of risk. In *Science, policy and risk* (pp. 13–30). London: Royal Society.

Omoto, A. M., & Malsch A. M. (2005). Psychological sense of community: Conceptual issues and connections to volunteerism – Related activism. In A. M. Omoto (Ed.), *Process of community change and social action. The Claremont symposium on applied social psychology.* Mahwah, NJ: Lawrence Erlbaum Associates.

Omoto, A. M., & Malsch, A. M. (2005). Psychological sense of community: Conceptual issues and connections to volunteerism – Related activism. In A. M. Omoto (Ed.), *Process of community change and social action. The claremont symposium on applied social psychology.* Mahwah, NJ: Lawrence Erlbaum Associates.

Omoto, A. M., & Snyder, M. (1995). Sustained helping without obligation: Motivation, longevity of service, and perceived attitude change among aids volunteers. *Journal of Personality and Social Psychology, 68*, 671–686.

Ott, K., & Döring, R. (2004). *Theorie und Praxis starker Nachhaltigkeit. Metropolis (Theory and Practice of Strong Sustainability).* Marburg: Metropolis.

Overstreet, S., et al. (1999). Availability of family support as a moderator of exposure to community violence. *Journal of Clinical Child Psychology, 28*, 151–159.

Pacelli, D., & Marchetti, M. C. (2007). *Tempo, Spazio e società, La ridefinizione dell'esperienza collettiva.* Milano: Franco Angeli.

Palumbo, M., & Garbarino, E. (2006). *Ricerca sociale: metodo e tecniche.* Milano: F. Angeli.

Paton, D., & Bishop, B. (1996). Disasters and communities: Promoting psychosocial well-being. In D. Paton & N. Long (Eds.), *Psychological Aspects of Disaster: Impact, Coping, and Intervention.* Palmerston North: Dunmore Press.

Paton, D., & Johnston, D. (2001). Disasters and communities: Vulnerability, resilience, and preparedness. *Disaster Prevention and Management, 10*, 270–277.

Paton, D., Millar, M., & Johnston, D. (2001a). Community resilience to volcanic hazard consequences. *Natural Hazards, 24*, 157–169.

Paton, D., Smith, L., & Millar, M. (2001b). Responding to hazard effects: Promoting resilience and adjustment adoption. *Australian Journal of Emergency Management., Autumn*, 47–52.

Patterson, J. (2001). Resilience in the face of adversity. *School Administrator, ERIC, 58*, 18–24.

Patterson, J. M. (2002a). Understanding family resilience. *Journal of Clinical Psychology, 58*, 233–246.

Patterson, J. M. (2002b). Integrating family resilience and family stress theory. *Journal of Marriage and the Family, 64*, 349–360.

Patterson, J. M., & Garwick, A. (1994). Levels of family meaning family stress theory. *Family Process, 33*, 287–304.

Peacock, W. G., & Ragsdale, A. K. (1997). Social systems, ecological networks and disasters: Towards a socio-political ecology of disaster. In W. G. Peacock, B. H. Morrow, & H. Gladwin (Eds.), *Hurricane Andrew: Ethnicity, gender and sociology of disasters.* London: Routledge.

Pelanda, C. (1981). *Disaster and sociosystemic vulnerability.* Disaster Research Center. Retrieved from http://dspace.udel.edu:8080/dspace/handle/19716/440.

Pelling, M. (2003). *The vulnerability of cities: Natural disasters and social resilience.* London: Earthscan Publications.

Peltu, M. (1988). Media reporting of risk information: Uncertainties and the future. In H. Jungermann, R. E. Kasperson, & P. M. Wiedemann (Eds.), *Risk communication.* Dortmund: Kernf orschungsanlage.

Penner, L. A. (2002). *Dispositional and organizational influences on sustained volunteerism: An interactionist perspective.* Tampa: University of South Florida Press.

Penner, L. A., & Finkelstein, M. A. (1998). Dispositional and structural determinants of volunteerism. *Journal of Personality and Social Psychology, 74*, 525–537.

Penner, L. A., Fritzsche, B. A., Craiger, J. P., & Freifeld, T. R. (1995). Measuring the prosocial personality. In J. Butcher & C. D. Spielberger (Eds.), *Advances in personality assessment: Vol. 10.* Hillsdale, NJ: Lawrence Erlbaum.

Perrow, C. (1984). *Normal accidents: Living with high risk technologies.* New York, NY: Basic Books.

Perry, R. W. (2006). What is a disaster? In H. Rodríguez, E. L. Quarantell, & R. R. Dynes (Eds.), *Handbook of disaster research* (pp. 1–15). New York, NY: Springer.

Peters, R. G., Covello, V. T., & McCallum, D. B. (1997). The determinants of trust and credibility in environmental risk communication: An empirical study. *Risk Analysis, 17*, 43–54.

Pfefferbaum, B. et al. (2004). *Executive summary: Community resilience mini-summit: Developing community resilience for children and families*, 24–25 March, National Child Traumatic Stress Network Los Angeles.

Pfefferbaum, B., et al. (2005). Building resilience to mass trauma events. In L. Doll, S. Bonzo, J. Mercy, & D. Sleet (Eds.), *Handbook on injury and violence prevention interventions*. New York, NY: Kluwer Academic.

Pfefferbaum, B., et al. (2007). Building resilience to mass trauma events. In L. Doll, S. Bonzo, J. Mercy, D. A. Sleet, & E. N. Haas (Eds.), *Handbook on injury and violence prevention*. New York, NY: Springer.

Pfister, C., & Summematter, S. (2004). *Katastrophen und ihre Bewaeltingung. Perspektiven und Positionen*. Berne: Haupt, Berner Universitaet schriften.

Phillips, B. D., et al. (2010). *Social vulnerability to disasters*. Boca Raton, FL: CRC Press, Taylor and Francis Group.

Pimm, S. L. (1991). *The balance of nature?* Chicago, IL: University of Chicago Press.

Plate, E. J., & Merz, B. (2001). *Naturkatastrophen Ursachen – Auswirkungen – Vorsorge*. E. Schweizerbart'sche Verlagsbuchhandlung (Naegele u. Obermiller).

Plodinec, M. J. (2009). *Definitions of resilience: An analysis*. Oak Ridge, TN: Community and Regional Resilience Institute.

Prati, G. (2006). *La resilienza di comunità*. Retrieved from http://emergenze.psice.unibo.it/pubblicazioni/index.htm.

Prati, G., & Pietrantoni, L. (2009). *Resilienza di comunità: definizioni, concezioni ed applicazioni* (pp. 9–25). XII: Psychofenia.

Prince, S. H. (1920). *Catastrophe and social change*. New York, NY: Columbia University.

Quarantelli, E. L. (1978). *Disasters: Theory and research*. Thousand Oaks, CA: Sage.

Quarantelli, E. L. (1982). What is a disaster? An agent specific or an all disaster spectrum approach to socio-behavioral aspects of earthquakes. In B. Jones & M. Tomazevic (Eds.), *Social and economic aspects of earthquake*. Ljubljana, Yugoslavia and Ithaca, New York: Institute for Testing and Research in Materials and Structures, and Program in Urban and Regional Studies, Cornell University.

Quarantelli, E. L. (1990). Conceptualizing disasters from a sociological perspective. *Mass Emergencies and Disaster, 7*, 243–251.

Quarantelli, E. L. (1993). Community crises: An exploratory comparison of the characteristics and consequences of disasters and riots. *Journal of Contingences and Crisis Management, 1*, 67–78.

Quarantelli, E. L. (1995). *Emergent behaviours and groups in the crisis time of disasters*. Preliminary Paper. University of Delaware, Disaster Research Centre.

Quarantelli, E. L. (2000). Emergencies, disaster and catastrophe are different phenomena. Preliminary Paper #304. University of Delaware Disaster Research Centre.

Quarantelli, E. L. (2005). *Catastrophes are different from disasters: Understanding Katrina*. Retrieved from http://understandingkatrina.ssrc.org/quarantelli.

Quarantelli, E. L., & Davis, I. (2011). *An explanatory agenda for studying the popular culture of disasters (PCD): Its characteristics, conditions and consequences*. Newark, Delaware: Disaster Research Centre.

Quarantelli, E. L., Lagadec, P., & Boin, A. (2006). A heuristic approach to future disasters and crises: New, old and in between type. In H. Rodriguez, E. L. Quarantelli, & R. Dynes (Eds.), *The Handbook of Disaster Research*. New York, NY: Springer Verlag.

Quarantelli, E. L., & Tierney, K. J. (1979). Social climate and preparation for sudden chemical disasters. In E. P. Lewis, L. D. Nelson, D. W. Scully, & J. S. Williams (Eds.), *Sociological research symposium IX*. Richmond, VA: Department of Sociology, Virginia Commonwealth University.

Quarantelli, E. L., et al. (1981). *Sociologia dei disastri: storia, teoria e ricerca*. Gorizia: ISIG.

Quennet, G. (1999). *La catastrophe, un objet historique?* Paris: Hypothèses.

Quinlan, A. (2003). Resilience and adaptive capacity: Key components of sustainable socialecological systems. *IHDP Update, 2*, 4–5.

Rapizza, S., & Held, M. (2006). *Voluntary action Italy*. Brussels: European Volunteer Centre.

Rappaport, J. (1977). *Community psychology: Values, research, and action*. New York, NY: Holt, Rhinehart and Winston.

Raymond, C. A. (1985). Risk in the press: Conflicting journalistic ideologies. In D. Nelkin (Ed.), *The language of risk*. Beverley Hills: Sage.

Reason, J. (1990). The contribution of latent human failures to the breakdown of complex systems. *Philosophical Transactions of the Royal Society B: Biological Sciences, 327*, 434–475.

Renn, O. (1992). Risk communication: Toward a rational discourse with the public. *Journal of Hazardous Materials, 29*, 465–519.

Resilience Alliance. Retrieved November 9, 2009 from http://www.resalliance.org/576.php.

Resilience Alliance. Retrieved September 25, 2006 from http://www.resalliance.org/1.php.

Richardson, G. (2002). The metatheory of resilience and resiliency. *Journal of Clinical Psychology, 58*, 307–321.

Rip, A. (1985). Experts in public arenas. In H. Otway & M. Peltu (Eds.), *Regulating industrial risks*. London: Butterworths.

Rodriguez, H., Quarantelli, E. L., & Dynes, R. R. (2006). *Handbook of disaster research*. New York, NY: Springer.

Ronan, K. R., & Johnston, D. M. (2005). *Promoting community resilience in disasters: The role for schools, youth and families*. New York, NY: Springer.

Rosa, E. A. (1998). Metatheoretical foundations for post-normal risk. *Journal of Risk Research, 1*, 15–44.

Rose, A. (2007). Economic resilience to natural and man-made disasters: Multidisciplinary origins and contextual dimensions. *Environmental Hazards, 7*, 383–398.

Rosenthal, G. (2004). Biographical research. In C. Seale, G. Gombo, J. F. Gubrium, & D. Silverman (Eds.), *Qualitative research practice* (pp. 48–64). London: Sage.

Rosenthal, U., Charles, M., & Hart, P. (1989). *Coping with crises: The management of disasters, riots, and terrorism*. Springfield, IL: C.C. Thomas.

Sapirstein, G. (2006). Social resilience: The forgotten dimension in disaster risk reduction. *Jamba Quarterly Bulletin of the African Centre for Disaster Studies, 1*, 54–63.

Savadori, L., et al. (1998). Percezione del rischio: esperti vs non esperti, Estr, Archivio di psicologia, neurologia e psichiatria, LIX, 3/4. Milano: Vita e Pensiero.

Scanlon, T. J. (1982, April–June). The roller coaster story of civil defence planning in Canada. *Emergency Planning Digest.*

Schnaiberg, A. (1980). *The environment: From surplus to scarcity*. New York, NY: Oxford University Press.

Schneiderbauer, S., & Ehrlich, D. (2004). *Risk, hazard and people's vulnerability to natural hazards: A review of definitions, concepts and data*. Brussels: European Commission-Joint Research Centre (EC-JRC).

Schneiderbauer, S., & Ehrlich, D. (2006). Social levels and hazard (in)dependence in determining vulnerability. In J. Birkmann (Ed.), *Measuring vulnerability to natural hazards – Towards disaster resilient societies*. Tokyo: United University Press.

Schultz, T. (1972). *Human resources (human capital: Policy issues and research opportunities)*. New York, NY: National Bureau of Economic Research.

Schutz, A. (1974 ed. 1932). La fenomenologia del mondo sociale. Bologna: Il Mulino.

Severi, S. F. (1996). Le ordinanze della Legge n° 225/92 sulla protezione civile. Milano: Giuffrè.

Shalev, A. Y., & Errera, Y. L. E. (2008). Resilience is the default: How not to miss it. In M. Blumenfield & R. J. Ursano (Eds.), *Intervention and resilience after mass trauma*. New York, NY: Cambridge University Press.

Simmel, G. (1903). The metropolis and mental life. In G. Bridge & S. Watson (Eds.), *The Blackwell city reader* (p. 2002). Oxford and Malden, MA: Wiley-Blackwell.

Simmel, G. (1995). *Le metropoli e la vita dello spirito*. Roma: Armando (ed. or. 1903).

Slovic, P., Fischhoff, B., & Lichetenstein, S. (1985). Characterizing perceived risk. In C. H. C. Kates & J. X. Kasperson (Eds.), *Perilous progress: Managing the hazards of technology*. Boulder, CO: Westview Press.

Smith, G. (2009). *Application and evaluation: What approaches are currently being used to asses resilience?* University of North Carolina at Chapel Hill. Retrieved from http://www.resilientus.org/wp-content/uploads/2013/03/Gavin_Smith_1248902597.pdf.

Smith, A. O., & Hoffman, S. M. (1999). *The angry earth: Disaster in anthropological perspectives*. London: Routledge.

Smith, A. O., & Hoffman, S. M. (2002). *Catastrophe and culture: The anthropology of disaster*. Santa Fe, NM: School for Advanced Research Press.

Sonn, C., & Fisher, A. (1998). Sense of community: Community resilient responses to oppression and change. *Journal of Community Psychology, 26*, 457–472.

Stallings, R. A. (1990). Media discourse and the social construction of risk. *Social Problems, 47*, 473–498.

Stallings, R. A. (2002). *Methods of disaster research*. Newark, DE: International Research Committee on Disasters.

Stallings, R. A., & Quarantelli, E. L. (1985). Emergent citizen groups and emergency management. *Public Administration Review, 45*, 93–100.

Starr, C. (1969). Social benefit versus technological risk. In R. Chalk (Ed.), *Science, technology, and society: Emerging relationships*. Washington: American Association for the Advancement of Science.

Thomas, W. I., & Znaniecki, F. 1958 [1918/1920]. *The polish peasant in Europe and America Volumes I and II*. New York, NY: Dover.

Tierney, K. J. (2003a). Disaster beliefs and institutional interests: Recycling disaster myths in the aftermath of 9–11. In L. Clarke (Ed.), *Terrorism and disaster: New threats, new ideas: Research in social problems and public policy*. New York, NY: Elsevier.

Tierney, K. J. (2003). *Conceptualizing and Measuring organizational and community resilience: Lessons from the emergency response following the September 11, 2001 attack on the World Trade Center.* Preliminary Paper #329, University of Delaware Disaster Research Center.

Timmerman, P. (1981). *Vulnerability, resilience, and the collapse of society: A review of models and possible climatic applications*. Toronto: Institute of Environmental Studies, University of Toronto.

Tobin, G. A. (1999). Sustainability and community resilience: The holy grail of hazards planning. *Environmental Hazards, 1*, 13–25.

Tobin, G. A., & Montz, B. E. (1997). *Natural hazards: Explanation and integration*. New York, NY: Guilford Press.

Tobin, G. A., & Whiteford, L. M. (2002). Community resilience and volcanic hazards: The eruption of Tungurahua and evacuation of the Faldas in Ecuador. *Disasters, 26*, 28–48.

Toennies, F. (1887;1912; 2005; Gemeinschaft und Gesellschaft. Grundbegriffe der reinen Soziologie), *Gemeinschaft und Gesellschaft. Abhandlung des Communismus und des Socialismus als empirischer Culturformen.* Wissenschaftliche Buchgesellschaft, Darmstadt.

Toennies, F. (1979). *Comunità e società*. Milano: Edizioni di Comunità (ed. or. 1887).

Tousignant, M., & Sioui, N. (2009). Resilience and aboriginal communities in crisis: Theory and interventions. *Journal of Aboriginal Health*. National Aboriginal Health Organization (NAHO), Organisationa Nationale de la Sanité Autochtone (ONSA). Retrieved from http://www.naho.ca/jah/english/jah05_01/V5_I1_Resilience_03.pdf.

Tremblay, M. A. (2006). The key informant technique: A non-ethographic application. In M. Palumbo & E. Garbarino (Eds.), *Ricerca sociale, metodo e tecniche*. Milano: Franco Angeli.

Turner, B. L., II, et al. (2003a). A framework for vulnerability analysis in sustainability science. *Proceedings of the National Academy of Science, 100*, 8074–8079.

Turner, B. L., et al. (2003b). Illustrating the coupled human–environment system for vulnerability analysis: Three case studies. *Proceedings of the National Academy of Sciences of the United States of America, 100*, 8080–8085.

Tversky, A., & Kahneman, D. (1974). Judgment under uncertainty: Heuristics and biases. *Science, New Series, 185*, 1124–1131.

UNISDR, WMO (2012). *Disaster Risk and Resilience.* Thematic Think Piece, Un System Task Team on the Post 2015 UN Development Agenda.

United Nations International Strategy for Disaster Risk Reduction (2005). *Hyogo Framework for 2005–2015: Building the Resilience of Nations and Communities to Disasters, and United Nations Interagency Secretariat of the International Strategy for Disaster Reduction (UN/ISDR). 2004.* In *Living With Risk: A Global Review of the International Strategy for Disaster Reduction (UN/ISDR).* United Nations, Geneva, pp. 16–17.

Van Dillen, S. (2004). Different choices: Assessing vulnerability in a South Indian village. In *Studien zur geographischen Entwicklungsforschung, Band 29.* Saarbrucken: Verlag fur Entwicklungspolitik.

Villagrán, J. C. (2001). La Naturaleza de los Riesgos. In *un Enfoque Conceptual. Serie: Aportes para el Desarrollo Sostenible, CIMDEN, Guatemala.*

Violanti, J. M., Paton, D., & Dunning, C. (2000). *Posttraumatic stress intervention: Challenges, issues and perspectives*. Springfield, IL: Charles C. Thomas.

Von Winterfeldt, D., & Edwards, W. (1984). Patterns of conflict about risky technologies. *Risk Analysis, 4*, 55–68.

Von Winterfeldt, D., & Edwards, W. (1986). *Decision analysis and behavioral research.* Cambridge, UK: Cambridge University Press.

Voss, M. (2008). The vulnerable can't speak. An integrative vulnerability approach to disaster and climate change research. *Behemoth – A Journal on Civilisation, 3*, 39–56.

Voss, M. (2010). Resilienz, Vulnerabilität und transdisziplinäre Katastrophenforschung. In A. Siedschlag (Ed.), *Jahrbuch für europäische Sicherheitspolitik 2009/2010.* Baden-Baden: Nomos.

Voss, M., & Wagner, K. (2010). Learning from (small) disasters. *Natural Disaster Hazards* Online First. Retrieved from http://www.springerlink.com/content/36k1300085616280/fulltext.pdf.

Wagner, H. J. (2004). *Krise und Sozialization Strukturale Sozialisationtheorie.* Frankfurt am Main: Humanities Online.

Walker, B. et al. (2004). Resilience, adaptability and transformability in social-ecological systems. *Ecology and Society, 9,* Art. 5. Retrieved from http://www.ecologyandsociety.org/vol9/iss2/art5.

Waller, M. (2001). Resilience in ecosystemic context: Evolution of the concept. *American Journal of Orthopsychiatry, 71*, 290–297.

Walsh, F. (2006). *Strengthening family resilience.* New York, NY: A Division of Guilford Publications.

Waugh, W. L. (1996). *Disaster management in the US and Canada: The politics, policymaking, administration and analysis of emergency management.* Springfield: Charles C. Thomas.

Waugh, W. L., Jr., & Tierney, K. (2007). *Emergency Management: Principles and Practice for Local Government (2a edition).* Washington, DC: ICMA Press, International City Management Association.

Weber M. (1981 ed. or. 1922). Il metodo delle scienze storico sociali. Torino: Einaudi.

Wilches-Chaux, G. (1993). La Vulnerabilidad global. In M. Andrew (Ed.), *Los desastres no son naturales*. Bogotá: La Red – Tercer Mundo Editores.

Wildavsky, A. (1991). *Searching for safety.* New Brunswick, NJ: Transaction.

Wisner, B., et al. (2004). *At Risk, Natural Hazards, People's Vulnerability and Disasters.* Trowbridge, Wiltshire: Routledge, Taylor and Francis Group, printed in Great Britain by The Cromwell Press.

Wolin, S. J., & Wolin, S. (1993). *The resilient self.* New York, NY: Villard Books.

Yates, J., & Stone, E. (1992). The risk construct. In J. F. Yates (Ed.), *Risk taking behavior.* London: Wiley.

Zimmerman, M. (1983). Methodological issues in the assessments of life events: A review of issues and research. *Clinical Psychology Review, 3*, 339–370.

Zimmerman, M. A. (1999). Emprowerment e partecipazione della comunità. *Animazione Sociale, 2*, 10–25.

Zimmerman, M. A. (2004). *Empowerment theory & adolescent resilience.* Oral Presentation at the Conference of European Association for Research on Adolescence, Portugal.

Italian Laws on the Issue of Civil Protection

Circolare 30 settembre 2002, n° 5114, Presidenza del Consiglio dei Ministri, Dipartimento della protezione civile: Ripartizione delle competenze amministrative in materia di protezione civile.
D. lgs 17 agosto 1999, n° 334, Attuazione della direttiva 96/82/CE relativa al controllo dei pericoli di incidenti rilevanti connessi con determinate sostanze pericolose.
D. lgs 31 marzo 1998, n° 112, Conferimento di funzioni e compiti amministrativi dello Stato alle Regioni ed agli Enti locali, in attuazione del capo I della L. 15 marzo 1997, n° 59.
D. lgs. 100/2012 Decreto-legge n. 59 del 15 maggio 2012 convertito dalla legge n. 100 del 12 luglio 2012: disposizioni urgenti per il riordino della protezione civile.
D.P.C.M 12 aprile 2002, Costituzione della Commissione nazionale per la previsione e la prevenzione dei grandi rischi.
D.P.C.M 12 dicembre 2001, Organizzazione del Dipartimento della protezione civile.
D.P.C.M 13 febbraio 1990, n° 112, Regolamento concernente istituzione ed organizzazione del Dipartimento della protezione civile nell'ambito della Presidenza del Consiglio dei Ministri.
D.P.C.M 18 maggio 1998, n°429, Regolamento concernente norme per l'organizzazione e il funzionamento della Commissione nazionale per la previsione e la prevenzione dei grandi rischi.
D.P.C.M 2 marzo 2002, Costituzione del Comitato operativo della protezione civile.
D.P.C.M 28 marzo 2003, Dichiarazione dello stato di emergenza in relazione alla tutela della pubblica incolumità nell'attuale situazione internazionale.
D.P.R. 6 febbraio 1981, n° 66, regolamento di esecuzione della Legge 8 dicembre 1980, n° 966.
L. 24 febbraio 1992, n° 225, Istituzione del servizio nazionale di protezione civile.
L. 8 dicembre 1980, n° 966, Norme sul soccorso e l'assistenza alle popolazioni colpite da calamità.
L. 9 novembre 2001, n° 401, Conversione in legge, con modificazioni, del decreto legge 7 settembre 2001, n° 343, recante disposizioni urgenti per assicurare il coordinamento operativo delle strutture preposte alle attività di protezione civile.

Web Source

http://demo.istat.it.
http://ec.europa.eu/echo/civil_protection/civil/prote/mechanism.html.
http://ricostruzione.regione.marche.it.
http://www.commissarioperlaricostruzione.it.
http://www.disastercharter.org.
http://www.disastermanagement.it.
http://www.economypoint.org/l/lidpar.html.
http://www.ispro.it.
http://www.iss-en.org.
http://www.labonne.org.
http://www.massemergencies.org.
http://www.norme.marche.it.
http://www.osservatoriosuldoposisma.com/molise/molise.
http://www.oxfordjournal.org.
http://www.protezionecivile.gov.it/jcms/it/terremoto_um.wp.
http://www.protezionecivile.it.
http://www.regione.molise.it/WEB/grm/sis.nsf.
http://www.ricostruzione.regione.umbria.it.
http://www.socialresilience.ch.
http://www.sociology.org.
http://www.trauma-pages.com.
http://www.vigilidelfuoco.it.

Index

B. Lucini, *Disaster Resilience from a Sociological Perspective*, Humanitarian Solutions in the 21st Century, DOI 10.1007/978-3-319-04738-6,

MIX
Papier aus verantwortungsvollen Quellen
Paper from responsible sources
FSC® C105338

If you have any concerns about our products,
you can contact us on
ProductSafety@springernature.com

In case Publisher is established outside the EU,
the EU authorized representative is:
Springer Nature Customer Service Center GmbH
Europaplatz 3, 69115 Heidelberg, Germany

Printed by Libri Plureos GmbH
in Hamburg, Germany